Tantric
Love
Letters

On Sex & Affairs of the Heart

Tantric
Love
Letters

On Sex & Affairs of the Heart

Diana Richardson

BOOKS

Winchester, UK
Washington, USA

First published by O-Books, 2012
O-Books is an imprint of John Hunt Publishing Ltd., Laurel House, Station Approach,
Alresford, Hants, SO24 9JH, UK
office1@o-books.net
www.o-books.com

For distributor details and how to order please visit the 'Ordering' section on our website.

Text copyright: Diana Richardson 2011

ISBN: 978 1 78099 154 2

A CIP catalogue record for this book is available from the British Library.

Design: Stuart Davies

Cover Art Artist: Anna Amrhein, Kuppenheim, Germany
www.Anna-Amrhein.de

Author Photo: Shobha, Sicily.

Printed in the USA by Edwards Brothers Malloy

CONTENTS

In memory of Beloved Shai
Your fragrance remains in the sound of music

Acknowledgements

My warm hearted thanks to the many people that have written to me over the years. I have enjoyed and valued the personal connection, as well as your questions, observations, experiences and insights. My special thanks to those of you who have contributed the letters selected for this book, and for allowing me to publish them. All the names and identifying details have been changed so as to ensure your personal privacy. To Ela and Simone, my appreciation for your kindness and generosity in helping me sort and select the letters. To Anna, thank you so much for your beautiful heart art that appears on the cover. To Raja, my eternal gratitude to you for your profound part in 'the work', for your inspiration, and for your love and lightness of being.

Introduction

Tantric Love Letters is a unique, interesting, and informative collection of authentic letters from people who have begun to look at sex from a 'new' perspective and bring about a 'change' in their way of making love. This personal correspondence is made available in order to encourage and support those people who have already embarked on a sexual enquiry, as well as to inspire or motivate others to begin exploring other dimensions of sex right away.

On the surface, the sexual realm feels to be particularly personal and individual. The question may well arise "How can the sex life of somebody else have any relevance to me?" The reality is that we are more similar to each other than we actually realize or appreciate - a fact that has become increasingly clear and obvious to me during my many years of teaching. This underlying truth means we can without doubt use the experiences of others to guide, help and support us to grow in love and understanding.

Sex is not given to us as a haphazard or random force that is subject to a person's chosen whims, goals, expectations or fantasies. The truth is that human sexual design is very precise and carries a deep intelligence in its roots; and sex has a higher potential beyond its reproductive or fun and entertainment function. Sex is a door that can lead to a step in human evolution, and not only to human reproduction. It is by changing the actual 'how' of sex that results in the quantum leap. Sex with 'heightened awareness' has a direct, positive and lasting impact on well-being and personal evolution. Sex 'rightly' employed is an empowering force that brings self-assurance and clarity, balances mood swings, enhances creativity, as well as significantly elevating the vibration of love within and around you.

And the by-product of this 'shift' is that the many sexual difficulties, relationship problems, personal insecurities and performance pressures commonly experienced spontaneously tend to evaporate. Love and harmony is re-created with extraordinary ease. There can be no higher endorsement to the value of making some kind of a 'change' in our sexual behaviour than these revealing facts alone!

The Letters

The letters that appear in this book are selected from an archive of several hundred letters that I have received, mostly by e-mail, from people living in many different parts of the world. Each person expresses in their own way the benefits of viewing or having sex from a fresh perspective. These letters also disclose the wide range of far reaching positive, healing, integrating and uplifting effects that accompany a change in the 'style' of sex.

Ever since January 1993 when I initially started to teach couples, and even more so since 1999 following the publication my first book, there has been a growing wave of affirmative response that continues until this day. The many insights and experiences of others have further served to corroborate that which I myself have experienced. To me this resounding 'yes' is the crystal clear echo of nature, confirming that such is nature's way, and according to her wishes.

Tantric Love Letters is definitely *not intended as a comprehensive sexual guide,* even though sexual advice is frequently given. A full sexual re-orientation and explanation is to be found in my earlier books.

Please note that all names and identifying details of contributors have been changed to ensure personal privacy. Should any similarity exist between a randomly chosen fictitious name and anyone else's personal circumstances, this is pure coincidence.

The Chapters

The letters are very loosely sorted and assembled under one of the following five umbrellas: Chapter 1: Positive Resonance & Response; Chapter 2: Relationship Themes; Chapter 3: Emotional Aspects; Chapter 4: Sexual Subjects; Chapter 5: Special Issues. Sometimes the theme of one letter will also appear as an issue in a another letter under a different chapter heading, but this level of overlapping is unavoidable. Chapter 3 on Emotional Aspects begins with a short introduction to the subject of emotions and feelings. The other four chapters do not require any special introduction as the chapter titles speak for themselves.

Usually the incoming letters are followed by my reply, but in several cases where the letter is a 'personal report' or a 'personal statement', my response is not always included. This is especially true in Chapter 1 on Positive Resonance & Response.

The Contributors

The people who have written to me fall into a few categories. Some I have met personally through their participation in one of the seven day residential Making Love Retreats for couples that I have been leading together with my partner Michael for the last twenty years. Other people have read one of the books and immediately put theory into practice by trying out some of the suggestions, and then afterwards have written sharing their insights and experiences. Some readers, even without any direct or personal experience, write expressing their appreciation because the information and orientation on sex simply has the ring of truth to it. Sometimes people write to me about their sexual problems on the advice of a third person - a friend, a therapist, or a counselor. And others with sexual problems search on the Internet and end up on our web site, and write asking for advice. In two instances where reports of personal experiences were pasted up on an American Internet forum, I took the liberty of turning them into a letter format.

In previous books I have used the personal experiences of others to support and endorse a new sexual vision. However, all of the personal sharings and reports that appear in this book, with the exception of one letter only, are published for the first time. In a few instances I have slightly amplified my reply for readers who may be less familiar with my approach.

The Approach

The human body contains a subtle inner design that is essential to know about because it enables us to honor our creator, and live our full sexual potential. The human body can be seen as a replica of the earth, with a magnetic North and South Pole. Like the earth, the body is similarly surrounded by and infused with a magnetic field. Each and every single human body is 'magnetically' conceived, as microcosm of the macrocosm. The body carries two energetically opposite poles that can be imagined as similar to a self-contained 'inner magnet'. One pole is located in the genitals, and the other pole is found in the heart. Because these two poles are of opposite polarity there exists the inherent potential/capacity for energy, vitality and potency to flow, circulate, stream and expand through and beyond the body.

On this subtle magnetic level male and female bodies are fundamentally different. They are equal forces, but they are also opposite forces. In this way man can be imagined as a magnet standing upside down, with the poles reversed. And it is exactly this basic incongruity and lack of similarity that makes male and female units highly complimentary and compatible. When the opposite poles of two magnets come into each other's presence there is a strong attraction, and energy flow within the individual magnets, as well as between the magnets. And the surrounding magnetic field is amplified. And these happenings take place without actually 'doing' anything. It happens naturally and spontaneously due to their innate properties and the proximity of the magnets in relation to each other.

Similar types of magnetic responses are possible within our own bodies, and between our bodies. Integrating and aligning ourselves with our significant 'magnetic' arrangement enables bodies to produce states of ecstasy and blissfulness. All that is required is our co-operation with the body and attempting to create an atmosphere that invites such higher experiences. Thus it is really a matter of having the right information in hand and a willingness to extend our sexual horizons.

There are two responses in particular that I have heard from people countless times over the years, words that touch me each and every time. Many say that they already 'intuitively knew' the information, but they did not trust themselves sufficiently to honor it. The second is that people report a deep sense of 'arriving home' in themselves for the very first time. These examples alone are persuasive enough, in that one shows that the knowledge already rests within our bodies, and the other points to its integrating and empowering effects. *Tantric Love Letters* is a way of sharing a wide range of personal experiences that can serve as encouragement to initiate or deepen a life-changing enquiry into sex.

Previous Books

My first book was written in 1996 and published in 1999 with the title *The Love Keys – A Unique Guide to Love and Sexual Fulfillment.* In 2004 it was republished as *The Heart of Tantric Sex* – with the same subtitle. This initial book is a comprehensive sexual reorientation that presents the basic 'Love Keys' in depth.

I have since written several other books, two as co-author with my partner Michael. However the basic view of and approach to sex does not change, it runs as a constant thread throughout. Instead, there are a number of windows through which the sexual experience can be viewed, where each outlook is valid and unique. *Tantric Orgasm for Women* is from the female perspective and informs woman of the higher potential that lies in the power of relaxation, receptivity and femininity. Likewise, the later companion book, *Tantric Sex for Men – Making Love a Meditation,* is viewed from the male angle, and informs man of ways to develop his innate potential and male authority by becoming 'present' to himself and woman in sex.

Alongside the importance of having an informed approach to sex, there is another basic requirement for harmonious love relationships – to have an understanding of the crucial distinction between 'feelings' and 'emotions'. These words are used interchangeably, however in reality feelings and emotions are physically and psychologically very different experiences. Knowing how to identify the difference imbues you with the power to 'protect' and sustain your love. In each book a chapter is devoted to this all-important subject. However, in the book *Tantric Love – Feeling versus Emotion, Golden Rules to Make Love Easy,* the information on how to distinguish between these two 'states' is removed from its sexual context, and elaborated into a comprehensive book, with the intention of making the information more accessible.

In my most recently published book *Slow Sex – The Path to Fulfilling and Sustainable Sexuality*, sex is viewed through the window of yoga and the existence of powerful universal metabolic enhancers. Embracing certain qualities - for example awareness and relaxation - can transform life from its very roots upward.

All of our books speak to the fact that in nature there exists a form and style of sexual communion between man and woman that is simple, sweet, spiritual, innocent, and fulfilling. A way that generates love and for which human beings are intrinsically designed. And such is the case whether a person knows it or not, or whether they choose to act upon it (by co-operating with their inner design), or not.

When we understand our sexual selves, we feel more in charge of our lives, more relaxed, more grounded, more centered, more confident. Love lies in our hands because we become capable of consciously creating love, nourishing love, and sustaining love. Sexual communion with 'intelligence' at its base has the power to spontaneously propel sex toward its higher vibration of love.

Glossary of Terms and Expressions

Below is a compilation of terms and expressions sometimes used in the course of the correspondence. The clarifications given below are simple and brief, and given solely with the intention of providing a few signposts to someone who is not so familiar with the territory. These explanations are not comprehensive and anyone wishing to understand the information and guidelines at a deeper level is directed to our previously published books.

Conventional sex: traditional style of sex where the energy is habitually built up to a climax/peak. Tends to be a short act because of high levels of excitement/tension.

Goal/orgasm oriented: ahead of the present moment, more focused on the next penetration because it takes you closer to the goal. General direction/intention is to reach an end, to 'come' or 'finish'.

Stimulation and excitement: the basic requirement to build up and reach a climax. Usually involves rubbing or friction of genitals, effort and tension.

Mechanical: where the movements in sex are repetitive, machinelike, unconscious.

Discharge of energy: the downward flow of energy/tension that accompanies the peak/climax. The energy is dispersed; it is not contained in the body.

Hot sex: sex where the temperature increases, built up to reach the climax. Using stimulation, sensation, and excitement as the way to get there.

Sexual conditioning: the inherited patterns of sex that are unconsciously absorbed from the society and make us have sex in a certain way, as in 'conventional' sex.

Sexual deconditioning: a process of using the awareness to challenge the inherited sexual habits that repress the life/sex energy.

Tantra/tantric sex: style of sex where there is no particular direction/goal/effort, it can unfold over many hours. The climax is not the point. It is an option. Energy can also be 'contained'. The habit of climax is reduced or abandoned.

Cool sex: style of sex where the temperature is kept intentionally low so that a person remains more present, in the here and now, not concerned about orgasm.

Awareness: the basis of tantric sex – to being more conscious and paying attention to what you are doing, and as you are doing it; avoiding being mechanical or going on automatic.

Present: attention is focused (in a relaxed way) on the very moment that is taking place, the actual here and now experience.

Sensation: where the stimulus tends to be more from an external source, or on the periphery of one's body, increases excitement and desire. Too much sensation can lead to eventual loss of sensitivity.

Sensitivity: where the stimulus/relaxed focus lies more within the inner realms a person. Receptivity to and perception of the subtle fine cellular movements in the body tissues that make up the 'inner world' of the body.

Receptivity: through being 'present' intrinsic capacity to receive, to absorb, to contain, to embrace, and to nourish life.

Dynamic: through being 'present' intrinsic capacity to convey, to flow, move, to channel, to radiate, to give life.

Containment/non-ejaculation: where ejaculation is neither controlled nor repressed, but where the sexual temperature is kept in the cool zone, and through less excitement/stimulation ejaculation is effortlessly kept at bay.

Magnetic intelligence/qualities: the human body similar to a 'magnet' with two poles, genitals and heart. Inbuilt capacity to circulate subtle refined energies within and between bodies.

Positive pole: body parts from which energy is raised or awakened. Woman/ breasts and nipples, man/area of the perineum.

Negative pole: places where energy is received. Woman/vagina, man/heart.

Perineum: small coin-sized muscular knot lying directly in front of the anus in man and woman.

Soft penetration: option of entry into woman without the need for erection.

Deep penetration: when erection is present to remain in the depths of the vagina instead of moving in and out.

Lubrication: almond oil for example, and suggest that it is used every time.

Scissors/side position: position where man lays on his side, woman lies on her back, and the legs are interlaced in scissor-style. Brings genitals into proximity.

Healing/purification: when awareness and relaxation are introduced into sex many old tensions or memories or pains spontaneously move out of the system, and in different ways.

Feelings: like sadness, love, pain, joy, that arise in the moment, and should be shared and shown.

Emotions/emotionality: feelings that are *not allowed*, kept in and repressed. Stored in the system and become toxins that then turn into negativity.

Symptoms of emotion: indicators that signify emotion e.g. disconnection, cannot look a person in the eyes, blaming, arguing, complaining.

Low-grade emotions: like a low-grade infection, where a person feels continually in a subtle state of disconnection, a bit blue, or slightly depressed.

Afterwards is your teacher: noticing how you 'feel' after sex, then evaluating this in relation to what you did during sex, and then being self-guided by the outcomes.

Meditation: simply relaxing into the here and now. Being with the genital connection as a center point for the awareness.

Blissfulness/ecstasy: a state of feeling oneself as pure vital energy, where boundaries dissolve, timelessness, immense peace and harmony.

Chakra: energy center, or "wheel" of which there are many in the body.

Kundalini: energy/vitality/life force lying coiled and dormant at the base of the spine (often likened to a snake), that is ultimately designed to rise.

Love keys: guidelines to increase awareness in the body moment by moment.

Tools not rules: tantric sex is not a technique with rules. Guidelines to use and experiment with in order to transform sex into more conscious experience.

Osho: spiritual master and mystic from India. Early 1970's he spoke in particular on tantra and the transformation of the sexual energy into a meditative energy.

Barry Long: spiritual master from Australia who produced revolutionary talks called *Making Love - Sexual love the divine way*, in the early 1980's.

Chapter 1

Positive Resonance & Response

1. The combination of love and spirituality is really fulfilling
2. Shown me a way of light through life
3. I am tantra!
4. Experiencing the intelligence of my penis
5. Changing our approach to sex has changed our lives
6. Our bodies started with tantra by themselves
7. Transformative aspect of this form of lovemaking
8. The heavenly effect of relaxing my vagina
9. The most valuable help in my over 80 years of life
10. Learned and experienced things that saved our love
11. Old pains in the vagina dissolved within two weeks
12. A refinement on all levels
13. Awakening of my breasts and connecting to the earth
14. Sexual healing for my arthritis
15. Sex with no excitement is deeper than any excitement

1. The combination of love and spirituality is really fulfilling

Dear Diana,

My partner and I met you and Michael during a retreat at the beginning of 2010. What we received from you both gives us the opportunity to live together in a way I have always been dreaming of. I had no clue about the concept and no clue what I would have to change as a man, but I often felt the essence of inner life would be possible for us, and that was the 'vision' that led me to your concept and your retreat. It is not a linear devel-opment – neither as a couple nor as an individual – but we feel that the path we are following is an outstanding and delightful one. Your concept is like the dot on the 'i' of all that I have experienced so far. We see now how traditional sexuality has been limited and in the end how problematic it is, in many ways. Whereas spirituality without our loving sexuality is just not the right way for me – but the combination of love and spirituality is really fulfilling for both of us. The healing path between the two of us based on your concept creates something wonderful in us. Something that is very difficult or even not possible to develop on a pure individual path. It is the honor of a couple.

Love, Ralph

2. Shown me a way of light through life

Dear Diana,

I'm sure you receive millions of e-mails written to you and your partner Michael, just to thank you for your amazing and incomparable support to human beings who would like to make their lives full of love and meditation. I cannot resist doing the same because you have really improved the quality of my life and shown me a way of light through my life. So, thanks so much, guys, I will always keep you in my heart.

Love, Alexandro

Dear Alexandro,

We really appreciate receiving your warm and enthusiastic message and thank you for taking the time to connect with us. It is very encouraging to hear that our approach, as shared in our books, is of help and support in your life and love. What is especially touching is that you have had the capacity to turn words into reality through your sincerity and intelligence, and for this we are very grateful. **Each individual who moves into sex in a more conscious way is doing great healing for our beloved Earth.** Wish you much love and light on your journey.

Love, Diana

3. I am tantra!

Dear Diana,

You may get a lot of e-mails like the one I am about to write, however, my passion propels me to write it anyway. I read your book *The Heart of Tantric Sex* and experienced the beginning of tantra with my boyfriend at the time. The doors opened and I know tantra is the path for me. In fact, this sounds strange for me to say, I simply am tantra would be more true!

Love, Sylvia

Dear Sylvia,

Thank you so much for writing to me. It is truly wonderful to hear of your resonance and the insight that you are tantra is deeply touching. Indeed such is the truth. **Each individual is born tantric** and it is a blessing and a gift that you are able to recognize your essence. Best wishes to you each day.

Love, Diana

4. Experiencing the intelligence of my penis

Dear Diana,

In December of 2007 I invited my longest standing (laying) erotic partner to read your book called *The Heart of Tantric Sex*. Our 'love connection' had been dead for over 20 years. No ecstatic experience left, dead, dead, dead. We naturally, effortlessly started following the instructions in the book, inspired and transported by something in it, something new, loving, some energy, wisdom emanating from its pages. Low and behold, we spent the next two weeks in 5 to 9 hour sessions reaching a state so beautiful I wanted to stay there forever. **I had never understood why people called sex - 'making love'. And here we were making, within ourselves and between us, a tangible love energy.** My intelligent penis 'knew' when her vagina was open. It knew to stay cool, in that receptive state where *it* was guiding me, *it* knew when to penetrate and how, my heart would be in joy, my whole body would feel touched by her vagina, we would remain for hours in this glow, we would lose sense of time. A few times I felt her heart touching my penis from very deep in the vagina. She had not self-lubricated in decades; she had lost contact with the vagina, now *it* became alive. At some point she said, glowing in deep appreciation, love: "I feel like a woman for the first time in my life." I am writing to you in gratitude about this life-awakening experience.

Love, Joseph

5. Changing our approach to sex has changed our lives

Dear Diana,

For the coming year we wish you and Michael all the best and lots of love. Furthermore, we would like to tell you about our rich experience since your retreat in June 2009. To have been able to take part in your retreat makes us feel deeply thankful.

I (Anna), at 52, experience sexuality in a completely new way as a woman. Until then I could only intuitively sense what a fulfilling sexuality would feel like. Today I feel a tenderness and sensitivity in my husband that gives me a nourishing security in sexuality and also in my everyday life. I found the power to let go of my expectations completely and to make appointments for making love, to surrender completely to the present moment, to allow, to 'let everything happen' and to flow into the togetherness with my husband.

It's getting ever clearer to me that the alert awareness of the present moment has helped me to be open and truly receive. I was able to discover this too because my husband has learned not to always ejaculate, and he does this by slowing down his movements. So he has developed a very fine feeling for the moment. Everything begins to feel as if it's weaving into one divine body of golden light, a truly divine love!

To me it feels as if I am finally allowed to live. I am allowed to give love and I am also accepted as a loving being. I can feel how my husband can heal old patterns and 'hardness' in my vaginal tissue with his penis. **My 'rusted-up love', that could never surface, is finally freed up and that in turn heals my husband's old wounds and gives us power.** It is very impressive to realize that if we 'don't have time' to make love we fall back to old patterns, we lose patience more easily and we treat each other less gently and even argue.

I am so grateful to know you and through you be able to get to know love in a new way. With such love our 'ill world' could change – because loving people live in peace and care for their planet.

I, (Felix), a 54 years young man, had in the beginning a lot of resistance to let go of habitual ejaculation. Today I enjoy making love to my wife for 20-30 hours in a period of 3-4 weeks without ejaculating. I have learned to be fine and tender and to feel my penis very consciously so as not to ejaculate. This is exactly what fulfills my wife. And this fine consciousness has also had an effect on how I treat her in everyday life. We hardly argue anymore. She feels accepted and loved, she blossoms and she has become my beautiful, tender fairy.

I am also surprised by an incredible power and harmony that I feel in my body. I can feel this, for example, while playing tennis. **You would think I am 20 years younger. I also I would not want to miss the repeatedly returning wonderful feelings around and in my perineum and the knowledge that I can unite with my wife again and again.** This gives an incredible feeling of belonging together. I feel that she likes to receive me because I treat her well (and myself as well) and not only meet her in order to live out my urge to ejaculate.

At last I want to congratulate you and Michael on your new

men's book – *Tantric Sex for Men*. The numerous reports of personal experiences were above all very impressive and convincing. I also have the feeling that it will never become boring to make love in that more relaxed way that you teach. Again and again we are surprised the new things we are able to feel and experience.

In deep gratitude and love.

Anna & Felix

6. Our bodies started with tantra by themselves

Dear Diana,

I read both of your books *The Heart of Tantric Sex* and *Tantric Orgasm for Women*. Thank God! This year my husband and I will celebrate our 25th anniversary. I will turn 45 in July. I entered this union as a young and innocent girl and I was full of love. Being with him physically fulfilled me most of the time. I loved him! We had a strong mutual sexual attraction, and we slowly developed regarding techniques, positions and closeness.

I was a very emotional woman and in this paragraph I can certainly confirm the 'emotional' problems, and in the way that you describe them as well. We built a house, children came and daily routine began. Tensions built up. **We argued and later had 'reconciliation sex'. Afterwards the tensions in body and soul were reduced, but at the same time this strange feeling of discontent remained and began to grow anew.** It was like with most plants, if you prune them they grow even stronger. This way our minor problems became major problems. About seven years ago we wanted to separate for the first and last time. It was a separation I wanted even though I loved him. Somehow we managed to reconcile for the hundred thousandth time.

And then the success story of our partnership began. The moment came when I found my inner calm through yoga, meditation and books (also Osho's books). Yoga taught me 'to accept myself as I am', and how to focus my attention in the body. Through meditation I could contain the flood of thoughts that filled my mind. I learned to be more relaxed, tolerant and neutral. And who would have thought it possible, but all my relationships improved, of course also the connection to my partner. Suddenly I recognized a different dimension in his behavior, in what he said, in his opinions etc. Before, he had only been a scapegoat for my emotions – exactly as you describe it!

Then we began to experiment more in bed again. We started to have very slow sex and I don't remember who instructed whom. **It was like in slow motion. For some short moments we would also remain motionless. Afterwards we realized that this had been the most beautiful sex we had ever had!** We were more than happy. We were satisfied! An old word has been given a new meaning.

Soon afterwards I went on vacation alone. There I found your first book. I was spellbound. In it I found confirmation that our bodies by themselves had started with tantra. Exactly as you describe it so lovingly in your books! That's great, isn't it? I can confirm you and you have confirmed me. Doing it and then reading about it – this is much better than reading about it and then doing it. (Most books come to a person accidentally, your book, Diana, for sure came from heaven.) When I returned from vacation my husband picked me up from the train and we went for dinner and right away I read a few lines from your book out aloud to him.

Ever since then we have been practicing. We are far from reaching a 'universal melting'. I cannot see bursting shooting stars or the like. But I can report how beautiful our physical union has become for me since then. This is how it is now: **If we manage to get away from the conventional in and out movements of sex and be motionless, and I also manage to bring my consciousness from my mind into my body, then after a certain time a pulsation starts in the genitals.** It actually feels as if a 'second heart' is beating in the abdomen. Currently I feel this pulsation only from the abdomen to the knees. In your book you say that *it* can spread into the whole body. I have not yet reached this level. Nevertheless already now *it* is so beautiful and it is very intense and not only quiet. And all this happened without effort, just from motionlessness and relaxation.

Since then my whole approach towards sexuality has changed quickly and so much for the better. Only through the tantric practice am I now able to see solely the good, the natural (yes!), and the sacred in the physical, sexual union. *It* is given to us by God and we *all* come from physical union. *It* deserves highest reverence and loving care. Suddenly a much greater context opens up to me. Yes! Now I can love unconditionally and be a woman. Now I can open up and receive. Now I enjoy sex because it fills me with love and energy.

As we have only been practicing for one year we fall back to the old method now and then. My head and my belly, however, still remember how beautiful slow sex is. How easy it is to start the lovemaking with slow sex and then later stop the movement altogether! Because only from here the pulsation I like so much begins.

I just finished your second book *Tantric Orgasm for Women* and I will give it to my daughter (21) for a special occasion. I wish with all my heart that she is able to free herself again from the compulsive conditioning (that I taught her).

There is one more thing I want to say. I also read other books about tantra. Most of them are full of techniques and medical explanations. Diana, **you wrote an anthem to the soul!** And you gave our confused minds easily digestible food. My favorite books are those where I feel that I could have written them myself. I could indeed have written some chapters. With the others I let myself be guided by you in full trust. Please accept my cordial thanks. For your books, the openness, and your courageous work! In deep solidarity,

Love, Hillary

Dear Hillary,

I am so delighted that you have taken the time to write to me and share so beautifully your experiences and profound insights. Thank you very much. I find it truly wonderful that everything evolved through your own inner exploration, and without any goal, and confirmation of your experience arriving only later. **In my experience, like yours, tantric communication is a natural language when we are simple, conscious and aware in the body.** And in this sense every human being is born tantric, with the inbuilt capacity to be aware and blissful in sex. Thank you for your being. My heart is with you.

Love, Diana

7. Transformative aspect of this form of lovemaking

Dear Diana,

Your books have been truly a blessing and I simply can't put into words what a difference they have made in our lives and our relationship. We both noticed the difference the moment we started putting into practice your teaching and have begun to experience the transformative aspect of this form of lovemaking versus conventional sex.

Our roots are in this part of the world, specifically Central America and the Caribbean where women are still very much oppressed by a culture where machismo rules. There is so much that I would like to share with you and get to meet you personally or even better, attend one of your retreats. For the time being, just know that you definitely are making a difference.

Love, Lawrence

8. The heavenly effect of relaxing my vagina

Dear Diana,

Thank you for your book, *The Heart of Tantric Sex: A Unique Guide to Love and Sexual Fulfillment*. It has truly changed my life. The companion book written with your husband, Michael, *Tantric Sex for Men: Making Love a Meditation*, is as good, if not better. I gave it to my lover after I read it. I think I enjoyed the men's book so much because I felt like I was being sneaky and peeking in on some of the secrets of male sexuality! I even felt a bit aroused!

There is a concept in your book that in all my life I have never known about, heard about, nor ever tried. It involves relaxing your entire pelvic floor, especially while making love. As women, we are used to tensing up the vaginal walls during intercourse because we think it makes it more exciting for the man to have more friction (and because it helps us to orgasm). And if we relax, we think we will feel too wide or loose for the man. I wasn't sure that I could manage to do it.

But I tried it. And Lord have mercy! It is the most heavenly thing I have ever experienced. It sounds simple, but it isn't. It is something I have to consciously stay focused on so I don't revert to my old habits. I was going to try to describe the difference it makes for me while making love (and what my lover tells me happens to him), but I cannot put it into words. It is something you have to experience for yourself. But what happens is the vagina becomes so open and receptive and welcoming when you relax the pelvic floor that it gives the man a wonderful feeling of being fully accepted. And when you do this while making love, the woman starts to draw the man up inside her like a magnet. And when the man relaxes his pelvic floor, he is able to feel the sensations throughout the entire length of his penis. The penis stays erect, but soft enough to snake around and conform to the vagina. It almost seems to grow in length.

And when you are still, you can truly, truly feel the electricity passing between you and your lover. It just pulsates. There is no need for movement at times. And you go into somewhat of a trancelike state where you just stay in the moment and feel. If you start to think of something other than the here and now, you direct yourself immediately back to the present. And the juices just flow! **In the past, if I had tried to have intercourse for two hours straight, well, it just wouldn't have been able to happen. I would have been dry and raw and so sex would be over.** But I stayed extremely wet and welcoming and it had a profound effect on his penis. I'm pretty sure this is the first time my lover has ever stayed erect (in varying degrees) for that long of a time and without getting tired or feeling pressured.

There are so many aspects of this – the healing aspect, the energy aspect, and it's all so incredibly relaxing and magical and mystical and yet thrilling at the same time. Yes, lots of mumbo jumbo, but it is there and you can't deny it.

And one of the other great things (I believe it is from both the books and also from the separate book *Tantric Love – Feeling vs Emotion*) I took away was discovering the distinction between emotions and feelings, and what to do when you have emotions well up inside you that normally would/could turn into something not so pretty. When this happened, I did what you suggested and said, "I am emotional" and took responsibility right away, right then. Not later. I experienced how instead, when you do so right away, you are accepting all of the feelings as your own and not blaming your partner for the way you feel. These insights of yours really, really helped me last week. We were beginning to make love, but I couldn't stop feeling guilty for the sacrifices he makes to see me every week. And instead of just holding it all in and letting it make me feel sad and perhaps projecting it onto him, I just said it out loud and it felt so good. I was able to cry, get it out of my system, while he was able to tell me why I should *not* feel guilty, and then we moved past it and made wonderful love.

So, two wonderful books and there is also much gratitude in my heart for Marnia Robinson, author of *Cupid's Poisoned Arrow* on whose Internet forum I found your book information, because otherwise, I would never have had this life-changing experience. Blessings to all!

Love, Kelly

9. The most valuable help in my over 80 years of life

Dear Diana,

It is not easy for me to write about the things we heard and learned from you and Michael during the week. You already know that it took me quite some persuasion to agree when my wife suggested that we do the course with you. But I can honestly say that already during the course itself, and later even more so, I have come to be convinced that this course is among the most valuable help I have ever received in my life. And I have received a lot of help in my more than 80 years of life.

What has happened to me in the almost 12 months after meeting you? **We told you about our golden wedding anniversary that took place soon after the course. It truly was a spiritual and emotional highlight. Preparing for it through participating in your course, our relationship was strengthened.** Since then we have been able to deepen it further. We often spend time together; we ignore supposedly very important work and afterwards we feel much more refreshed and motivated to continue working. Alternating weekly, one of us is in charge of deciding about when to meet and how to meet, and what elements to include. When the motivation is high enough a semi-hard erection is possible and works for soft penetration (which we practice most of the time). We spend up to one and a half hours together. Most of the time I nap for a short while. Then we again trace the inner circulation of energy with the breath. This creates a very soothing and peaceful atmosphere. Also our general condition is very good. There are fewer headaches, less tension, more feeling of warmth, circulation etc. When I am away on long walking tours then we still have a fixed time for long distance daily contact, meaning that individually we lie down and each tries to connect the rhythm of the breath with the imagination of closeness and intimacy.

Love, Thomas (82 years)

Dear Diana,

Now it is my turn to describe how 'things' have been for me. Firstly, I want to sincerely thank both for all the good that Thomas and I were allowed to receive through you. As you know, first there was the book *The Heart of Tantric Sex* that encouraged us to participate in your seminar in 2005. The book alone had already changed many things. And then of course the seminar, our so-called honeymoon before our golden wedding anniversary. To get to the point: Our sexuality has become calm, relaxed and very joyful. We were given an incredible deepening and enrichment – imagine, at our age! This has a very positive effect on our everyday life.

Now I have also read your book *Tantric Orgasm for Women* with great interest and again I gained a lot from it. I will try to explain my questions, problems or difficulties to you. First there is the issue with presence. I have to bring myself back to the *here and now* again and again and I notice that I feel the energy flow very well when we are both fully present. It also happens, though, that Thomas falls asleep and I am suddenly fully present and feel like taking off. This is the case in the scissors side position that we use most of the time because of the softer erection.

As the erection is weak most of the time, I have difficulties to put the penis really inside me, so then the penis is just before the real doorway. Nevertheless, the meetings are pleasant for both of us. Does that mean that the energy is flowing even like this? Then I imagine how the penis grows and how it penetrates me very deeply. This also gives me a very good feeling. For both of us I wished it were true. Now I also feel my vagina very well and my breasts begin to live. How beautiful. The difficulties with the soft penetration are for sure also due to my uterine prolapse. It does not need surgery but it would be better if I had three hands. Even though we are still very flexible it is hardly possible to maintain the genital contact with a soft erection while changing positions.

Of course, just a change helps to stay present, even if we lose the contact and have to put the penis in the vagina again. Thanks to the 'new' relationship with Thomas I am of course in a very good mood. May this be an insight into our joys and difficulties.

Love, Manuela (78 years)

Dear Manuela and Thomas,

Thank you so much for taking the time to write and share your experiences. You are a rare couple having the insight to begin a sexual exploration at this stage of life. Through your great steps you are giving the rest of us tremendous encouragement by showing us what is possible, for which we thank you. **Certainly what you are experiencing bears testament to the fact that sex does not need to fade out in the later years, as is very common.** And also it is wonderful to hear that you are discovering that sexual communion is generating more love and vitality and happiness, as individuals and as a couple.

As you have observed, presence is a key, and on some days it will be better than other days. What to do? That is why it is recommended to do something physical or active before you make love, such as short dance or some quick exercises, and energize yourselves as individuals. When the body is inwardly alive it is much easier to hold the awareness in the body, rather than drift off into thought or sleep. When one person is more present than the other, then you can use your presence to draw the other into the situation. Or if one person falls asleep it is no big deal either because your own inner world of sensitivity and delight will usually continue.

To answer your question, yes, the energy will flow, even when the contact between penis and vagina is slight. Using your imagination is a very good tool to deepen this connection, just as you are doing, and I am pleased to hear that you feel its satisfying effect. It is understandable that you would both prefer a stronger erection, but for sure it is better just to relax into a simple acceptance of 'what is'. With this supportive attitude energy is free to flow where and how it wants. When there is a tension with 'what is', as in if there is a weak erection, then inwardly there is a deep disconnection from the experience. It becomes like an inner fight that makes the body tense and unreceptive.

You may well find that after a time erection per se will lose its significance. In many ways the emphasis on erection is because of the conventional hot sex approach, and the sexual imprints we receive. In reality erection does not really matter. You will forget about it! Certainly this is what happened to me because of the possibility of entering without erection, or soft penetration. I just lost the 'idea' of erection; the thought did not cross my mind anymore. When erection was there it was there, when it was not there, it was not there. There was no longer any evaluation. But this shift happened with time and I am sure that with continued practice the same will happen for you.

What you certainly can do is to bring your breasts (as woman) increasingly into the picture, resting more with your awareness in the breasts and nipples than in the vagina. Doing this will expand your body energy and also cause a resonance in the vagina, making her more receptive and vital. In this way you can contribute to the general atmosphere, rather than thinking about erection. In the same way a man brings his awareness to the base of his penis – the perineum area.

What is helpful before you make love is to lie down together, separate and side-by-side, for ten to twenty minutes. You bring attention to your breasts/nipples, and Thomas brings his attention to his perineum. Remember, these are the positive poles. Doing this is a very good preparation because it will begin to polarize your energies in relation to each other.

I really like the way you have decided to take alternate weeks to be 'in charge' – it really makes life so simple and relaxing. I have tried that too. It saves a lot of discussion about what to do, when and how. And to enjoy/value both experiences – one of having the responsibility to decide/choose, and the other experience of accepting/surrendering to someone else's decisions/choices. Both are equally important.

I deeply appreciate you both for your intelligent, courageous and curious hearts. Best wishes for each and every day.

Love, Diana

10. Learned and experienced things that saved our love

Dear Diana,

In March 2008 my husband and I were in the Making Love Retreat and there we learned and experienced things that have saved our love. Even though before we did not feel that our love was threatened. Looking back now, however, knowing about the tremendous difference, I see how desperate our sex had been. How unloving we had been and how much we had searched for each other. I am sure that our love would have died and also our relationship would have broken up eventually.

After one week of making love in a more conscious way it was as if the fog between us had cleared, and full of surprise, I realized that my husband was standing in front of me, looking at me tenderly. Before I had not been able to see him any more.

In the first three months I was sometimes a little bit afraid that we could fall back into our old program, lose ourselves again. But that cannot happen. If we are only the least bit aware we notice what is good for us and what is not.

For sure you receive a lot of letters like this from grateful couples and they probably all write the same things. For sure every one says: You have changed my life. You have saved my love! All the same, risking that you will hear this for the hundredth time, I want to tell you some things that changed so much by our making love:

- I am always ready to make love; more often even than my husband.
- I love to be allowed to be passive; it is so pleasurable for me to surrender to him completely. Before my husband took my passiveness as indifference and was hurt. Now he loves it as much as I do and sometimes he even corrects me a bit when I become too 'active'. This way I also learned to accept him as he is. No matter if he is passionate and hot

or calm and motionless I love to receive him, to be there for him, without reining him or making him small or giving him guilty feelings.

- *I have never again had any inflammation of the vagina. Before I had it with wearying regularity every two or three months.*
- I still do not experience peak orgasms but sometimes I have small, extremely unexpected orgasms, sometimes happening out of complete calmness, that feel as if a few cells explode in my genitals.
- And sometimes I feel as if suddenly an enormous space opens in me as if stepping into a cathedral. I suppose this is what you describe in your books as valley orgasms.
- Making love connects us anew again and again. When we make love in the evening we would love to stay awake the whole night and cuddle.

Love, Kirstin

11. Old pains in the vagina dissolved within two weeks

Dear Diana,

My wish to come to your retreat with a partner was realized this year in June when I came with my new boyfriend. It was a beautiful week, from the content, from the ambience and from the deep relaxation we experienced. Until then for years I always had pains in the vagina when I made love to a man. Suddenly I would cry out because it hurt me so much. My gynecologist explained to me that a muscle in the vagina is tense. There was nothing to do about it. This pain caused me to lose my joy of sex.

In the week in June during the seminar with you two times the tears were running down heavily while making love. Old pains were melting. **The pain in the vagina dissolved within two weeks after the seminar. First it was weaker, and then it was suddenly gone. What a relief!**

I also have had images and been in heavenly worlds where I was shown by heavenly beings what and how the divine essence of life is. It is not easy to put in words. This vision of 'divine essence of life' or 'nectar of life' had an explicit color and consistency that is difficult to describe – namely off-white to beige, a nebular fluent aura. In the vision it was flowing out of a spring and was dividing into two streams. In the meantime, I have several times recognized a light flowing off this cream/off-white aura during lovemaking. It only emerges after one and a half or two hours of lovemaking and I guess it is identical with the orgasmic energy.

For my boyfriend and me lovemaking has become something very important. Even though I'm much more connected with your impulses than he is. But it doesn't matter, even if he doesn't want to practice, we still find ourselves on a level that nourishes us and makes us very happy. I bow to this energy. **Isn't it wonderful that I am over fifty years old and I have never in my life felt so much as woman, and lovemaking has never been as fulfilling as it is now.**

Love, Jutta

Dear Jutta,

Thank you very much for your loving gratitude and for your beautiful and profound sharing. What a blessing that you have found a way to enjoy making love again. Especially impressive is how quickly the pains in the vagina disappeared. It is a joy and encouragement to hear of personal experiences after the workshop, and how a simple more conscious body approach is healing and creates many qualitative shifts in a person's life. I am touched by your receptivity and sincerity, and for allowing my words and way into your being. And for the fertile soil that you prepared for these seeds through your many years of personal exploration.

Wishing you the joy of love each day.

Love, Diana

12. A refinement on all levels

Dear Diana,

The seven days with you and Michael were a refinement on all levels. We spent a few days in Berlin afterwards. We retreated to our hotel suite to make love several times a day. This had the effect that we moved through the big city in a much more centered and relaxed way than usual.

Back at home we bought the book *The Heart of Tantric Sex* which now inspires us almost every day, answers questions and resolves smaller misunderstandings. Our making love has become slower, more energetic, less 'sportive' (smile). **Even though I did not have physical problems with the conventional style I often felt 'energetic-emotional' disharmony before, during and after sex. This also caused these 'strange moods'.** Since we are now making love more slowly and more consciously, I definitely feel inwardly more balanced. More and more often I find myself in a relaxed, flowing and at the same time powerful state that I have always been looking for but not been able to find somewhere else that easily and naturally. My partner and I are connected more deeply and softly in the heart while on the level of our personalities there is more space between us and this again reduces the emotions.

This is our short feedback four weeks after the retreat. In any case we will continue this joyful research and we again deeply thank you for your absolutely essential inspiration!

Love, Martina & David

Dear Martina & David,

Thank you for your beautiful message and sharing your experiences and insights since the week we spent together. It is truly moving to hear how you have taken the tantric message deeply into your hearts and feel so many empowering and uplifting effects. Wishing you both a loving and wonderful summer.

Love, Diana

13. Awakening of my breasts and connecting to the earth

Dear Diana,

Especially these days I have been thinking of you very often because I started to do something that you recommend for all women – to meditate regularly on their breasts. I never realized how important this was, even though you say it time and again. I have been using your and Michael's guided meditation *MaLua Light Meditation for Women* on the breasts to support me – and now finally (I am so happy!) I can feel the energy flowing very softly through my body and also down into my legs. I almost started crying when I felt it for the very first time! **It was my heart's wish to feel my legs, to root myself in the earth, to really be able to 'stand' and tell my truth in an authentic way with integrity.** And I know deep inside: now I can heal, now my nervous system will be balanced. I always had these trembling legs (like after a shock) when I felt that now I would have to speak and tell my truth. I can feel so much energy and power in my body and I urgently need to be grounded well. Now this starts to become reality in my life. I am so glad and grateful that I had and have you as my teacher. May you and your work be always blessed with love and grace.

Love, Maria

14. Sexual healing for my arthritis

Dear Diana,

"It is arthritis!" That was the doctor's diagnosis a few years ago when he examined my aching finger joints. Something inside of me strongly refused to accept this final diagnosis. I asked myself: This may be the diagnosis but what is the cause? In the numerous courses I attended in Polarity, Focusing, Trauma,

Rhythmic etc. I had learned to consciously focus on the inside. I understood the interplay of introjection and projection. The more I focused on my inside the more I was able to trust myself, my being, and my abilities grew. I felt the difference between being in love and love. The heart connection to my partner became stronger.

Despite all this knowledge and extensive experience I became more and more distant from my long-term life partner – physically and therefore often in all areas. A slow process began. It seemed to be a paradox. I felt a deep love for him and the very intimate wish for connection and still my vagina became drier, sore and tighter. Lubricants did not help.

Is this part of the menopause? But then, why do some women have a fulfilling sexuality up until old age? It had to be my fault! I could still have an orgasm with oral stimulation but a big part of my being felt neglected and after such meetings I felt empty, often isolated and sad. This could not be it. I knew that there had to be 'more'. Our physical encounters and contacts happened less and less frequently. We have so many things in common. I feel his love – but what's the matter with me or us? Why does my sensuality fall by the wayside so much? We were often on an emotional roller coaster; we even got to speak about separation.

Then one day I had lunch with a friend of mine. She mentioned this wonderful Making Love Retreat week in Switzerland. It had been one of the most beautiful holidays she had ever spent with her husband! I started to listen attentively and asked for the address. This could be the rescue measure we needed! When she is so happy about it and shines so much it has to be a long-lasting seminar. First my husband was resistant to follow my wish but after several talks his attitude luckily changed from skepticism to acceptance. I had learned to deal with the pain in my fingers. When I protect my borders (physical and psychological) and take good care of myself my fingers feel healthy even with their deformation.

I learned in your tantra seminar that my so-far conditioned sexuality is very closely connected to these borders. It happened during the second afternoon. We were in our bedroom lying next to each other in a meditative way without any expectations. We were like two beginners, trying what had been suggested to them. I felt the warmth of his soft penis in front of my vagina. The warmth increased and suddenly a current of energy 'shot' through my body from head to toe. Above all the energy of my heart and my whole torso widened, my arms and hands pulsated as if connected to an electricity grid. Tears of joy and gratitude ran down my face. We managed a soft penetration and I had two wonderful hours in an indescribably pleasing connection with myself, with him and with everything that is. The energy became calmer and streamed evenly upwards. I felt the circulation between us and it was wonderful when my partner said that something was drawing his penis upward, deeper into the vagina. I had exactly the same sensation. It was very soft, very tender and very exhilarating. This is healing. Sexuality that connects me to something greater, that nourishes me and makes me come to life.

I felt intensely that there is a connection between the painful fingers and my former sexuality, as well as different forms of violence, emotion and abuse. (Rheumatism is also said to be a result of pent-up fire energy and sexuality is our life fire.)

The setting of the tantra week is unique and profound. I would experience, understand or get a sense of something, and then the very next day your explanations in the sharing's and theory part always confirmed my own notions. **Thank you very much for this sensitive teaching and your loving support. We gained from your incredible presence, respect and the good pinch of humor. To see you as a couple and as tantra teachers gives a big healing impulse.**

My partner at one point was very challenged by his boundaries and his old wounds. He became desperate and even

35

considered leaving the retreat. It was too much for him. Then, the same night, we did the exercise to relax the solar plexus. I had only just touched my partner and already his tears started to flow and he felt the painful parts getting softer and more integrated again. For him this was the 'key to be able to continue'. When I asked him after the seminar if he would do it again he answered with a heartfelt yes, and we immediately registered for the next year!

Moving from overwhelming sensations (be it drumming or dancing for example) towards very fine and slow rhythms is often a completely new challenge for me. The world screams so loud that I am put off my stride. With the help of tantra this disturbance is happening less frequently because both poles are satisfied in a wonderful way. The conscious, tender and aimless way of being together is soul food and much more than the intensity we have had so far.

Often our being together also triggers 'healing pains' in the way you explain it. It is as if the issues (partly familiar) in the deepest layers of the cells come up (once again) and then leave forever. One day in particular when we were making love, I felt a tightening in me and in my vagina, and informed my partner that I was contacting sadness but did not know why or what it was. I asked him to stay were he was, if possible, and to pull back the penis a few millimeters (as you suggested), and to stay there inside me with awareness. My tears were flowing and then I thought I felt impatience arising in him. Understandable as we were still only able to do soft penetration and he had told me that he also would like to feel a full erection inside of me. Full of fear I asked: "Are you getting impatient?" and then suddenly the whole issue became visible. He said: "No, it is not impatience, right now I cannot tell what it is, it rather feels like helplessness regarding the situation." Then the whole pain flowed out of me. I was allowed to show all my sadness, fear and pain – what a liberating process. Both of us felt how the vagina became soft and relaxed. The energy moved and the connection got pleasurable. My beloved was still shining the next day and he said: "I did not have an orgasm, my penis was not fully erect and nevertheless I got a boost of energy like never before. Unbelievable!" The most beautiful feedback for me!

For me and increasingly also for my partner this respectful, present lovemaking is much more fulfilling than everything I or we have experienced before. Our partnership is revitalized through a new closeness, an openness and depth that we did not even experience in earlier times of strongly being in love. Our gratitude is immeasurable.

Love, Roxanne

15. Sex with no excitement is deeper than any excitement

Dear Diana,

I want to send you a deep, deep thank you for all the doors you opened, for the wonderful impulses and hints you have given me on my path of making love. I have such a wonderful time in making love (and far beyond, all the way into everyday life and work) with my girlfriend, we are touched and so happy about what is possible to experience without any excitement. We enjoy to the fullest. Not so easy to describe and still I am sure you understand anyway. Today we made love and for me it was the *very first time* without any excitement, zero, zilch. **Even though you say that sex without excitement is possible, I did not think that it could really be that way, and yet the experience went deeper than any excitement ever could take me.**

Amazing! So I continue again and again to harvest the fruits your words planted in my being. And I am very, very grateful!

Love, Sam

Dear Sam,

It is indeed a great shift when you have the awesome experience that there is a level of sexual exchange that is beyond excitement. Not against excitement but beyond it! Your experiencing this level of reality is truly a mark of your sincerity, staying on track over the years, listening, learning, and practicing. And so my appreciation and thanks are due to you too!

Love, Diana

Chapter 2

Relationship Themes

1. My addiction to hard sex is much stronger than his
2. My partner is not used to giving to a woman
3. My husband has fallen in love with someone else
4. New love and a new chance
5. I want to explore sex more than my husband
6. My girlfriend moved out and will not talk to me
7. We both want something better than we have
8. Can tantric sex help me reconnect with my girlfriend?
9. It is clear for me that I must separate
10. After some time of marriage, sex got unbearable
11. She's the woman I want to love and cherish with all my being
12. My girlfriend is afraid of trying a new way of making love
13. My wife has lost interest in sex since birth of our son
14. I do not feel like being intimate with my husband
15. Our personal discoveries based on your books

1. My addiction to hard sex is much stronger than his

Dear Diana,

I experience it being not very easy to overcome my old sexual conditionings. Interestingly this is much more so for me, than for my man, who is not a sex maniac at all. I am much more into sex than he is, and I feel both the desire to enter new spaces of 'sex in love', *and* to go on enjoying – yes I do enjoy! – 'hard' sex. I can witness it all objectively, but this does not help. **Really it is an addiction, and 'I' do *not* *want* *to* miss the feelings and states** involved. **It is hard to accept that my addiction to 'hard sex' is much stronger than my partner's,** who is happy to have discovered something new, although he is also still occupied with his own fears of not getting an erection without certain stimulation.

I feel very ashamed and hurt about his judgments about the hard sex we had before (and enjoyed, but he always experienced it as uncomfortable and shameful), and I have the feeling that I don't know how to meet him 'just as woman', not the bitch, the slave or whatever. I am afraid we may separate because our sex life falls apart, that he will not turn me on any longer, that my lust vanishes and then my life will be empty and without meaning etc.

I do see some light in the distance somewhere, and I know it is high time to look even more deeply to my conditioning, to learn and to go for something new. But I still want to be hot also, not only do what you suggest and have holy sex without arousal and climax. What to do?

Love, Cynthia

Dear Cynthia,

Thank you for sharing your experience and observations. Interesting that you can clearly see the conditioning and the strong hold it has over us. Just this seeing of it is already a shift, a loosening from the grip of habits and patterns. Things don't change overnight, but happen more in small steps, a subtle transformation that will take time and requires lots of making love. **The key is to make love with increased awareness, and that is all.** When you find/notice you are moving into sex that has a 'goal', start to do so with awareness, it is as simple as that. **You will notice when there is a goal in mind that the body gets hardened, tense and contracted, which localizes the sensations and intensity. When you get tight and narrow, you also become less sensitive and feel less.** So instead, look to see how you can get to your destination in a slow, easy and relaxed way.

Make it a dance, a play, relaxing along the way, less focused on the outcome or goal. *Any* inner relaxation will lead to increased sensitivity and waves of vitality expanding throughout your body, which can be very satisfying and touching. Simply be aware and attempt to move your body in a more conscious and 'soft' way as you build up into a climax – that is the way to go. When things do perhaps turn toward 'hard' sex, then 'watch' and observe yourself doing so, inwardly take a step back from the situation so that you are less identified with it.

Also important is to observe yourself after sex, how you feel as an individual, and also notice what is going on between you as a couple. Usually the focus is around the climax, and not much attention is given to the experience and feelings *after* sex. When you start to observe that the level and quality of love and harmony increases when you are more aware in sex, or have 'sex in love' as you so nicely put it, this will encourage you to move forward in your exploration. This aspect of 'how you feel afterwards' is the greatest teacher possible. You start to put thing together noticing a correlation between what you do, how you do it, and the after-effects. And in fact this how I taught myself. And do not be too short term with your 'afterwards' by which I mean watch yourself over several days, not just the few hours after sex. Take note of any mood swings or if you are getting 'emotional' and blaming or complaining, notice how 'loving' you feel toward yourself and/or your partner, and the level of harmony between you, and in your life in general.

I sense through your words that you have much insight and awareness of your situation, and awareness is the basis of transformation, so you are on track. It is an ongoing process, not something that happens instantly and overnight. **The sexual conditioning is very deep and in every cell of the body and psyche, and takes time to dissolve and lose its power and grip. Your love for sex is a great asset, and your quest can be to bring the light of consciousness to shine on it – regardless of what it is that you actually do. Changing the way you make love is certainly *not about rules*, what to do and what not to do, what is allowed**

and what is not allowed. This clinging to rules is technique and does not represent real transformation. Our approach is more a question of *how* you do something, and not *what* you do.

Yes, there is a deep fear of emptiness in most of us, so what you feel is understandable. All I can say is it is wiser to move forward into the unknown than to let the fear keep you in certain patterns. You will remember that during the retreat we said that "fear is the absence of love," and this means you need to work on love and not go with the fear or the absence. So in this sense, love is the direct medicine for fear – and the more you make love, and be more loving toward others, you will notice the fear begins to subside. So let there be a commitment to making love frequently and simply start out with the intention of remaining as aware as you can, for as long as you can, that's it. Even noticing that you are beginning to lose awareness is already an act of awareness. Just a few words of encouragement to you to keep exploring, enjoying, being curious and observant, and they come with my best wishes.

Love, Diana

2. My partner is not used to giving to a woman

Dear Diana,

Yesterday I shared a little bit with my partner what came up for me and which emotions pass through when we make love – very often I get angry and feel hurt because he is not present, has no erection, or if he has, he gets excited and falls back in the pattern of using my body and vagina to get more excited. Then my emotions of rejection follow, not getting what I need in terms of being touched and caressed in the way I like it, and of course the fear that I don't turn him on. All this happened Sunday night when we were lying in bed and for the first time I managed to stay as a witness to all these emotions and remain receptive and present nevertheless. It was a nice experience, although the next morning my old symptoms of candida infection showed up. This time I am more relaxed about it than usual because I am realizing that maybe this is part of detoxification and letting go of old memories, and is not coming through as real infection.

In our sharing yesterday my partner described himself for the first time honestly as somebody who is not used to giving in lovemaking, that it is still very new and often strenuous for him to take care of me and my own needs. He says he still does not feel much in his penis, which takes a lot of his energy and attention.

This makes me very sad; I realize that I always suppressed this insight: I do not have a lover who is very experienced in arousing a woman for her own pleasure, and not for his own pleasure. And yet I know that this insight is obviously also part of the way, of *our* way: **I have to learn to become more receptive and not to do and give all the time as I used to in my old role which was always pleasing the men and not really feeling my own needs and feelings. Incredible, how much I really believed I like and want hot and hard sex.** This is still hard to process – my body reacts in a positive way to this by some sort of cleansing (of the candida), and yet a little disturbing voice starts to get louder in asking if this is really true?

Love, Abigail

Dear Abigail,

Thank you for your sharing your situation, many things happening on different levels. To share what you feel is valuable in getting to know each other on a deeper level. As I see it, basically none of us have been taught about love, how to love, how to give, how to share, so often aspects of an individual will look very personal when in fact they are not personal at all. Instead they are collective issues, or male/female issues, or both, and all of them the by-product of zero education in love and loving. So instead you can use the situation with your partner to support and love each other back to a healthy balance of giving and receiving. As well as receiving through giving and giving through receiving.

As you become more receptive as a woman, this enables a man to give more easily. **Your receptive welcome creates 'space' for his energy to flow from his being; he is invited and received. So in this sense woman has much power in sex.** The more you can 'be' and the less you actively 'do', the environment around you and within you is transformed. Through becoming receptive, woman becomes a force, which draws man toward her. So there is a natural flow that is beyond any conscious effort, it's spontaneous. Our effort is to create the situation of femininity and receptivity, and all else will follow on.

My suggestion is you continue to make love regularly and concentrate on your own receptivity, and things will get easier. Even if you feel he is 'not present', rather focus on your own presence instead of looking at his shortcomings. It is quite normal for a man to have diminished sensitivity in the penis when he becomes less active in sex. But the fact is the more frequently you make love the more likely it is that your partner's sensitivity will return. His admitting to his inability to truly give to woman, or that he feels nothing, is part of his own transformation and finding his own deeper authority as man. So you will need patience and practice and I suggest that you don't be influenced by little voices that try to devalue your actual experience. Wishing you a loving summer.

Love, Diana

Dear Diana,

I am very confused at the moment about everything because it seems I am together with a man who simply is not as much attached to sex, or rather to lovemaking, as I am, and I *do* suffer from that. In my perception I have done what I can; I do my best to agree to *only* once or twice per week, I very consciously watch my patterns and program concerning sex, and yet: what remains is that I wish for more, that I am missing the closeness, the pleasure, the feeling of being wanted, that I am very often angry at him because I find it boring to just cuddle most of the times, if at all.

We talked so much about it, and my partner very quickly only feels pressure, while I see myself as really having been open for everything. Again and again inviting him to also open new doors for the subtle feelings in his body and experiencing sex in a new more conscious way, but he concludes basically that he simply does not 'want it' as often as I do.

Of course I do have to accept this because I really love him, and I don't want to separate. I want to make love with him, not *any* other guy, but I also feel restricted in my liveliness, pleasure and sexual energy which wants to flow more often. And I want it to flow with him. **This really gets more and more serious; I even have problems going to sleep, because nearly every night it is the same – he is tired, and I am longing for him. I don't show it any longer but I cannot sleep then and my mind starts going around and around.** We are stuck in our feelings of rejection and frustration and repression and anger on my side and probably pressure and lack of self-worth as man from his side. What to do?

Love, Abigail

Dear Abigail,

My heart goes out to you, loving your man, and also the sense of not being met on a physical level. And I understand your longing and disappointment. It is a delicate situation. In such cases I do feel, generally speaking, that very often the stresses and anxieties associated with survival consumes much of our vitality. And this affects our creativity and sexual interest. Also as humans we tend to live in our bodies in a very lukewarm way; we are quite mechanical and have limited awareness of the body at a deeper level. It is as if an inner fire has slowly gone out, and we are all a bit dead, much less sensitive and alive than is our potential. Our bodies are barely used in the daily routine; many of us are physically relatively passive. Our inner sensitivity needs to be awakened and this can be done through regular exercise and increasing the level of body awareness in simple things; how you sit, how you stand, how you drive, etc. will be a good beginning. But each individual needs to wish to enquire, it has to arise for themselves; they cannot be told that they have to do it. Instead of focusing on him and what he is not doing, you can create an environment that invites him and encourages his awareness.

I suggest that you start to move your energy in other ways, and take the focus off your partner. Through exercise or dance, for example, you can begin to feel the inner fulfillment of these activities. You can also work on your inner sensitivity and begin to meditate on your breasts for half an hour each day. Your feminine qualities will be encouraged and amplified. In these ways you can be less dependent on your partner. This also means that when you do actually get together there will be less pressure on him because you are more fulfilled and at ease. Bring the focus back to yourself and your body as much as possible. Cuddling presents you with a wonderful opportunity to dive into your inner realms. And you may also notice how a shift towards your own center can sometimes invite a spontaneous response or movement in your partner. Your own inner focus can have the power to draw him into the awareness and aliveness of his own body. So when you are lying together cuddling, don't think so much about what you are *not* getting, and perhaps getting emotional on a subtle level by inwardly complaining, but find how you can explore *yourself* in the given situation.

Turning inward is extremely nourishing, energizing and uplifting. And if you are more content with your own inner universe, and what it gives you, then your partner is more likely to turn towards you. Too many complaints and demands will push him away. When possible make love during the daytime, or the morning, when you partner is more likely to be fresh. Best wishes to you both.

Love, Diana

3. My husband has fallen in love with someone else

Dear Diana,

It is so hard to write and tell you that my husband has fallen in love with another woman. I am devastated. We have had such a beautiful time for so many years and things were improving too, especially since we started to change the way we make love. He cannot take the decision to leave his girlfriend, but at the same time he wants to start to work on our relationship. Again and again he says that love will decide how everything will go on. I get so emotional that I want to just finish the relationship with him. And I definitely don't want to make love with him, even though he wants to. I ask him how it will look practically when love decides? This is what he answered me in writing: "I think that love will have decided when both of us can completely say yes to this love and to ourselves as free human beings, and without dependence on expectations, norms and fears. This is a high goal, I know, but together we can try to get there. I think this path is worth the pain. I am also very desperate when I don't know how to continue but there is always a next step."

How shall I handle this situation? Does it make sense to wait then? I cannot feel inside myself what is the right thing to do. I really feel stuck and there seems to be no way out. How do I know when it's better to move on? I would like to have more contact to my inner voice.

Love, Irmgard

Dear Irmgard,

I am really sorry to hear you are experiencing challenges in your relationship, especially after all your years of shared love and deep experiences together. I have enjoyed you immensely as a couple the several times that we have met each other. Life has clearly presented you with an unexpected twist and turn, but these things do happen. And how we deal with them can make all the difference. What you do know for sure is that great love connects you and your husband. And because of the fact you have been exploring and transforming sex together for several years now, you have formed a completely new basis and foundation for your relationship. So you need to recognize and trust what you have created together.

If you do not 'know' what to do, then you don't do anything. Just wait and be with the situation. It is better not to make a decision, rather wait and let life unfold and then the next step will become clear. You will not have to decide anything because you will *know* what to do. This will help to get in touch with your inner voice. So the way through is to 'accept' what is happening, painful and difficult though the reality may be. To accept that the beloved is having an affair is one of the most heart-wrenching realities to face as a lover. The sexual force at times is 'magnetic' and where there is a certain level of ease, awareness and presence, there can be attraction. What to do? If he is able to take the keys he practiced with you and be conscious with the other woman, then for him this can an empowering and learning experience. And it happens, more often than not, that the man will return home in great love and appreciation of you.

The truth is the process is seldom easy. But all the same we have to do our best to use the awareness and maintain a perspective on the situation *and stay open*. And definitely watch the mind which is a star at winding you up and creating a storm of emotion, perhaps convincing you to take revenge in some way, tell him leave the house, or to make him suffer in some way. Stay where you are and continue your life and projects as best you can, focusing on your body and inner world.

The most important thing is to release all the feelings of grief and sadness that come up in you. And do so *as they rise*. Don't bury and avoid your feelings; you may even need to weep for some hours each day. This will keep you feeling fresh, soft and open. By doing this, when you do actually meet him face to face, you are not charged with the tension of any unexpressed feelings (emotions) that can easily cause negativity and disconnection. You will be more present, more vulnerable, innocent, sweet, available, and real.

Let him go in love, and tell him he can come home anytime he wishes. Be an open door and an open heart. You have to decide that you want love in your life instead of emotion. In this acceptance there lies a chance (but no guarantees) that he flows back to you in time, to the place where he feels truly at home. You will need to hold the space at your end as a woman, and not make decisions and give up on everything, your man, your marriage, right away. Give him a bit of space, let him do his thing, and wait. Any vulnerability that you are capable of bringing into the situation, lack of blame (acceptance), and allowing the feelings of insecurity, these qualities will serve to transform the space within you, around you and between you.

If you react and do not allow him home, or you do not want him to make love with you 'on principle' because he is making love with someone else, then you will get stuck in a certain 'emotional' frame. And this can affect the how the future unfolds. Emotion will prevent a fresh level of meeting in the present, because the past (emotion/unexpressed feelings), are being pulled into the present and disturbing the moment. The decision to handle the thing with awareness instead of going into emotional patterns or dramas can save your relationship. When we go again and again into unawareness and emotional reactions, there can be unfortunate consequences. When we move with awareness and love the outcome is likely to be more positive, growthful and uplifting.

One thing I have always found helpful is the understanding that we cannot possess or own another person; ultimately the other is free to live their own life. Sometimes the pain we feel comes from jealousy and possessiveness, and not from love itself. Love is tremendous insight, clarity, sensitivity, and awareness. If we truly love a person then we want the very best for them, unconditionally. If the experience is valuable for your partner then that is significant in terms of his life, and his growth. If you 'allow' your man to move with another woman, in my experience, he returns empowered. And therefore he will usually be in a greater position to love you. I also know it is not at all easy when confronted with the actual situation!

My very first tantric lover was very open to women and it was not always possible for him to keep our prearranged dates (for making love) because sometimes other invitations from women came his way! I was naturally very disappointed and upset but I also saw very clearly that I had a choice each time he reappeared on my doorstep. The question I found myself asking in that moment was always: Did I want war (as in drama and where have you been?) or love (as in hello, and let us get together without further words). I can only say that choosing for love each time saved me, and helped me to stay on the tantric track. I was learning and discovering something so valuable when making love with him, I was basically more interested in going for that, than going for the emotional drama. This I had definitely experienced (many times!) when previous lovers had been 'unfaithful'. I do feel today that if I had stood in my own way then, at that early stage of my exploration, I would not have been able to gain the overview and understanding that I now have.

I wish I could say something to make your passage easier but I know, from my own experience, that it has always been growthful. The danger is to cut him out of your heart and become hardened toward him, because doing this also hardens you and disconnects you from your own essence - which is love. If you can stay with love right now, stay in contact with your heart and love for him, in spite of the situation, this will be the very best for your now, and for your future, because future emerges from the now. The negative influences of emotion and the ego can easily harm love if you are not aware of them. My thoughts and heart are with you both.

Love, Diana

Dear Diana,

Thank you very much for your words of support and comfort. I can definitely feel how getting caught up in my emotions closes my heart and blocks my love for him. And really when I am honest, I do love him and I want him in my life, I do not want to unconsciously push him away. So you are right, I will have to pay attention to my feelings and not let them turn into emotions. I recognize that I have always had a deep fear of losing my man, and I guess this is the case with many women. So in that sense what I am dealing with is nothing new to me. It feels like, in some strange way, a form of healing for me. I see how I place my man in the centre of my life, instead of myself. I notice that in the moments when I stand in the centre, he moves toward me naturally and lovingly. I know that this process will make me more secure as a human being. And help me to develop the love for myself. I sometimes experience myself as only half a woman when my man is not around. Now is the time to feel myself whole, independently of man, whether he stays or goes. I sense that what I have learned in the years of making love in a more conscious way will stand me in good stead for any other love affair or relationship. I realize that what I have learned through being in a 'couple' actually has been a profound learning as an individual. I have new tools and understanding that I can carry forward with me day by day. Thank you for your help.

Love, Irmgard.

4. New love and a new chance

Dear Diana,

Since our first meeting and attending two seminars, a couple of years have passed. Eventually my partner and I decided to go separate ways, and today we are best friends but the sexual curiosity was missing. **We still love each other very much and we managed to separate in a way that was positive, without any blaming or negativity or emotion, and I am sure this was because of our tantric understanding and experience.**

In the beginning of December I met someone new. For me he is a fascinating man. Next to him I feel quiet, in harmony, and simple. He has never heard anything about bodywork, therapy, or anything like this. At the moment, I need a suggestion, a tip on how to continue. It is difficult for me to speak to him, especially to show him how I want to live my sexuality, how I want to be touched. Because I also want him to feel good and that he can live his sexuality. So I try to live conventional sex, to mix it with what I learned through the seminars. But this is so difficult for me. I lose myself very quickly and forget what is good for me. Last weekend I created the perfect drama. The needy, disregarded, unfulfilled child was present and in retrospect I realized that I was totally emotional.

I want to live with him because the feeling is right. Only sometimes I get desperate and I have the impression that we are living in two worlds. He would like to come to the workshop because he wants to understand. Is there a possibility to make emergency space for us? Or do you have an idea how I could convey to him what I need in a better way? So far we spent three vacations together. Then I do not have a problem. I can stay relaxed. I know that we have enough time to also satisfy my needs. There is enough time to build closeness etc. **In everyday life he works in shifts, mostly in the night and on weekends. Then we do not manage to spend much time together. I do not have enough time to create the closeness I need.** He works in a very boring sitting job, and he needs a lot of action afterward, which means he wants to be active, and go out – instead of arriving – which is what I long for. Besides this I have the feeling that we are speaking two languages: what he says does not correspond to what I feel. And when we talk about sex it gets especially difficult for me. As I write to you now, I realize that I need to stay even closer to my truth.

Do you have a suggestion how I can manage it with a 'normal' man? He has problems with erection. He will turn 40 this year and he does not want to speak about it. My feeling is that there are two men: one in the head and one in the body – the body one he does not like very much. The problem is that I like this body-man. If I try to speak to him he goes into his head. **He hates**

woman who speak in bed while having sex. It disturbs him. While I write it down I start to feel more loving toward him – it sounds crazy. I would be grateful if you have an idea how we could pass the time until we can participate in one of your workshops.

Love, Carolina

Dear Carolina,

I am so happy to hear that you have found a new man and a fresh opportunity to grow in love. And yes, it can be a challenge when you have some tantric experience and input, but your new partner does not. And to change the way of making love is not something you can force on a person; you have to wait until the interest or curiosity arises from their side. It is quite usual for men not to have any impulses to change the way they make love, because what they have experienced so far is all they know. And mostly men are happy with that. What a man really needs is a little taste, a flavor, or a glimpse of something different, in order to awaken his longing or curiosity.

The very good news is that through your attending our workshops, together with the experiences with your previous partner, you now have the awareness and insight on how to hold the present, and thereby create a tantric atmosphere around you and within you. Do not wait for the other person to do the same as you, or be the same as you. Instead, just do it by creating a spacious environment, relaxing into your being, alive in your senses, through awareness and presence. And in my experience, man will very naturally respond to this level of invitation and welcome. He too becomes simple and present. And this can take place without saying anything in words. As a woman, creating this atmosphere is especially easy because it is woman who is the receptive force, the container, the milieu, the space. Relaxing into your femininity, being here and now and not going for excitement and orgasm, will give you more authority and influence during sex because of the innate 'holding' power of the receptive force.

What is said during the retreats, and in the books, is that tantra is an individual journey not only a couple journey. **If you want more relaxation and awareness, then *you* start to be that. And through some special alchemy your partner will begin to follow you, because when woman truly receives, really only then can male energy begin to flow!** So in your situation and with your background there is a great deal of creativity possible, areas you can grow and expand into.

I suggest that when you make love you begin to melt into your breasts, be relaxed and do not build up excitement, stay present, eyes open, breathing deep and slow. If your man wants to build up excitement, you relax instead of participating. If he wants to have an orgasm, you relax and don't try and have one too. The more you can communicate or convey a new language through your body and using your awareness, the better. Use talking and explaining as little as possible - especially since he is sensitive to talking.

I am unable to arrange a place in the workshop in the next period of time, as they are fully booked. Perhaps you can read the books aloud to each other, so that you begin to have a common understanding and approach. The workshop is useful in terms of getting a quick download of information, but the real 'work' starts when you get home – making love regularly. So in this sense you are not at a disadvantage. Remember your strength lies in 'being in the awareness' and this draws the other person into the present. So you definitely have a situation of new love, new chance. In your hands you hold the possibility of a great adventure, one of exploring your feminine power that will make you more woman, love and light. On a daily basis meditate on your breasts for twenty minutes or so. Best wishes and blessings to you and your partner.

Love, Diana

Dear Diana,

Thank you for your words. I know that I should be more relaxed. This is something I want to learn. I notice that I always feel more concerned about what happens to the person next to me, and so easily I lose inner contact to myself. And also I need the courage to show who I am. I try to hide myself so as to avoid the possibility of being rejected or hurt. The part you write about the man is also helpful to me. Allowing myself to be myself, and to be with myself, and especially when together with my partner is a challenge for me. **My problem is that if I think that there is only this moment, then I want this moment to be perfect. There is a picture in my mind how this perfect moment should look. And this somehow blocks me.** I realize that I need to change and allow myself to try things out and experiment, and that there will be a next time and a next time for me to accumulate experience and learn. So it does require me to trust in life and in love, which is not so easy for me. To trust that there will be enough time, that the moment itself is perfect like it is, and that I don't have to act anything out to make it perfect, and that my partner is okay like he is. To be like this is much easier if I am not emotional. To recognize that I am emotional is very difficult. Because if I am emotional it means that I don't want to change, so there are big things to learn. Thank you for your answer. It's a good motivation and I feel I am on the right way.

Love, Caroline

5. I want to explore sex more than my husband

Dear Diana,

I am stuck in a hole and don't know how to go on. When we make love it is only for half an hour at most and afterward I am frustrated and I feel used. I believe that only I am working on myself and my husband is going back to old patterns. He does not do anything to reduce his level of emotions because he is convinced that he does not have any. He only wants to make love in a hard way. As soon as his penis is not erect anymore then making love is over for him and he dreams away. He does not like it when he is soft inside me; he only wants to be inside me if he has an erection. He says that I have to contract the muscles of my vagina because if not he does not feel anything and he cannot enjoy it. I also cannot be present in my body during making love.

The moment I try to talk about these things with my husband he feels attacked and withdraws. Meaning he gets emotional but he never wants to admit it. He does not work anymore, he retired last year, and we definitely have the time to do exercises or dance or meditation but he claims not to need it. I have the feeling everything depends on me and I cannot handle it alone. Sometimes during making love I have the feeling that he is demanding. I cannot talk about it with him because he feels hurt immediately. In spite of the fact that he says he is not emotional and does not need to exercise or move. I, however, think that if he learned to reduce his emotions or at least to recognize them we could take a step further.

I feel helpless and I do not know how to change the situation. Instead of enjoying retirement we are wearing ourselves out. What do you think about the situation and is there any special meditation that you could recommend to me?

Love, Patricia

Dear Patricia,

Sorry to hear about your difficulties. Yes it can be that one partner is committed to growth and transformation and the other partner is not really so interested. **Finally, I feel, the best thing you can do is to realize that you cannot change the other person. To do so is impossible. Interest in transformation cannot be forced on someone.** The way forward is to change yourself in subtle ways, to see what you can do within the limitations to make the situation more acceptable. For instance, one possibility is to let go of all the expectations and wishes that you have, especially around making love. Certainly to do this will be a disappointment for you, but in the circumstances you have to come back to yourself. Your focus is somehow more on your partner, what he is not doing. And as you observe, you yourself find it difficult to be present.

I often will say that tantra is first and foremost a commitment by an individual; it is not really a couple commitment. The individual comes first, and the couple comes second. So when/if you realize that you are alone in some way, then there are many ways of exploring yourself on your own: do breast meditation twenty minutes every day (the MaLua guided meditation CD recently published), daily exercises, relaxing the vagina and pelvic floor again and again during the day, attempting to be aware of your body in all your daily activities, your breathing, etc. If you enjoy some particular exercises, then do them, if you enjoy dancing, then dance! Don't wait for him. If there were one special meditation to suggest, then that would be to meditate on the breasts. But at the same time you can make everything you do a meditation by doing it with awareness. This is the tantra way, the tantra life.

It is good to be aware of your emotional state. And remember that it is often easier to see the other person's emotions than your own. **For sure now is not really the first time you have felt frustrated, disappointed or used in sex; it is bound to have happened before, so the way you feel now also relates to your past experiences too.** This view may help you to have more distance to the situation. If you find yourself complaining or blaming the other person for your unhappiness, then it is usually a sign of emotion. When this is the case, then do something active to release any backlog of emotion and unexpressed feelings. So you need to continually monitor yourself, and come back to yourself, finding access to your inner happiness. And you do have much happiness inside you already – you are a wonderful, sincere, and intelligent woman!

As long as you push your husband, he is going to (consciously or unconsciously) push back and resist in different ways. This implies that when you do come back to yourself, your partner then has the 'space' to make a move toward you. But you must not expect it from him. An important thing to be aware of is that pulling back and coming home to yourself *does not mean cutting off* (being emotional) from your partner. It means accepting him like he is, loving him as he is, and being happy that you have a way to be involved with yourself. When you start to love yourself this love radiates outward and becomes a great invitation. I hope these few words offer you some support.

Love, Diana

Dear Diana,

Thank you for your words, they helped me to feel more relaxation and trust in myself. I have been a bit emotional it is true, so I have been working on that level the last few weeks. And I feel much better. I have also been focusing on myself and on my own body, and that has been very beneficial. I feel much more content and self-contained. Not demanding love, but giving love. **The miracle is that after this shift back to myself, my partner suggested we make love, and we have been doing so quite often since then. I guess when I took the pressure off then, like you said, he would open up.** I can't tell you how beautiful my man looks the more he makes love in a relaxed way. All the folds and creases in his face have smoothed out, and he looks much younger and he shines. So much to discover, even as pensioners, and we feel fortunate to have a new vision about sex and love.

Love, Patricia

6. My girlfriend moved out and will not talk to me

Dear Diana,

I was so confident that we found a solid basis for ourselves and our future, however, my girlfriend started complaining about things that have existed already for a long time, e.g. that my son in his twenties is still living with us, and that my smaller children are leaving a mess everywhere when they return home to their mother. The mess was never that big, but finally my girlfriend was dissatisfied with everything and everybody. All my attempts to open her up and to find out what's wrong failed. She moved out of our apartment while I was away on a business and when I came back I found our rooms empty. **I have tried to get in touch with her many times but failed. She does not answer the phone and if I send email she answers that it does not make sense to talk because we never understood each other in the first place, and it will be the same if we talk again.**

I am totally confused and have no idea about what happened, and I would like to know what would be the best way to act in this situation. Of course I feel that it makes no sense to urge her, she will need some time to organize and to find herself. On the other side it is so hard for me only to work on an energetic level. I send her lovely thoughts every day with the invitation to her to open again, and to build up a basis for an open and respectful communication. But I also tend to call her and to urge her, well knowing that this can be counterproductive.

I would appreciate if you have any advice for me. What to do? How to do it? I am especially concerned about having the patience to wait until my girlfriend is willing to talk to me. My instinct tells me it will be a few months; however, this will be a long period of time to wait.

Love, Rudolph

Dear Rudolph,

I am sad to hear of disturbances in your love field. It is very hard when a partner moves out without communication, and is basically in a closed-down emotional state. Emotion makes it a delicate situation, in that it is usually better to give the person space to deal with and digest their reality, rather than to keep pushing to make contact. It is a hard one and you will need to be patient. You can only hope that the emotional phase soon passes, or your partner has insight into her emotional state, and she comes back to you with an open heart. **Sometimes there can be such an emotional accumulation from the past that a person finds it hard/impossible to track back to love in the present. Remember that other men lie in her past too, as sources of dissatisfaction or frustration, so**

what she is experiencing is not *only* **to do with you.**

In the meantime, I suggest that you be loving and gentle with yourself, finding ways to nourish yourself, and be in love with yourself. When you do decide to make contact with her, then be sure that you are not emotional in any way when you communicate or share. By that I mean that you are not complaining or blaming her about the situation, which can even come through in the tone of voice that you use. If you wish to invite her back into her life you will have to feel the invitation deep in your being and in your heart, as I am sure you do. And you will need to talk about yourself, and communicate your love and your longing, and then she is more likely to respond from the heart.

If emotion is floating about in you, and she hears it indirectly or directly, then easily the invitation is not experienced/heard as an invitation. So if you should feel some unresolved issues on the emotional level, some feelings that you need to feel and release, then it is probably a good idea to deal with these before you take up any contact. I can feel your sincerity and your deep love for your woman. I wish you the best and hope all evolves according to the wishes of your heart.

Love, Diana

Dear Diana,

I am deeply grateful for your taking the time and answering my message. In the meantime, I decided to give my partner the space she needs, although it is very hard for me not to call her and not to visit her in her office. I will work on an energetic level and send her love and peace and say that I will welcome her back if she decides to talk about returning to me. Even if we live apart, I can imagine continuing our relationship. She is the woman I have had the best life with and everything was really great.

By now I know about my contribution to her moving out. The last few weeks she complained that I do not value her, and after asking what her needs are regarding feeling valued she could not give me a clear answer. I assume there is something beyond anything she or I are aware of at the moment. I feel very sad about not being able to talk to her about her decision, and not to be able to say farewell to her in a respectful and peaceful way. In the meantime I started working on some childhood traumas that appeared during a meditation. I have lots of friends who are supporting me and I do not feel alone but enjoy my apartment, and it has a completely different clear energy now.

Love, Rudolph

Dear Rudolph,

Thank you for writing again and it is good to hear that you have support through your web of connections. It is a beneficial sign that childhood issues are clearing themselves, creating more space for love and light to flower within you. I feel the most significant and transforming aspect of your process the last months is that you have *stayed open*, and not gone into emotional reaction and distance.

You can be sure that your partner's feeling of not being valued is something that goes way back into her past, and probably it started in her childhood and with her parents or father. And she has probably had similar feelings of being undervalued in previous relationships too. So in this sense her emotional withdrawal is not only personal to you.

Yes, perhaps there were moments in which you did not value her, but the wound is much deeper than this. If there was no wound lying in the past she would have dealt with the situation differently, and her heart would have been easier to reach. Your capacity to stay present to what is, stay open in the heart in spite of rejection again and again, will definitely strengthen your male authority and male essence.

Love, Diana

Dear Diana,

It has been very difficult confronting the last six months, and until today my girlfriend has not been willing to talk to me. **However, a while ago I met a mature and self-aware woman and making love with her is like a dream. And I am able to**

make love with her in the tantric way so easily; we just fall into this space of the present. I also see and feel how all women are the same in their essence, the same sweetness, and the same shine of love in their eyes. We live in different countries so we arrange to stay together for several days and then we have to leave each other again for a several days or weeks. This is very thrilling because the longing for each other is growing steadily! Thank you for all your support to get clear with my situation.

Love, Rudolph

7. We both want something better than we have

Dear Diana,

I'm currently reading your book *Tantric Orgasm for Women* and find it utterly fascinating. My husband and I have been together for twenty years this month and the last few in particular have been extremely difficult. I'm in a lot of pain, Diana, and **sometimes I find it difficult to pick up your book because I know that what I'm reading rings so true in my heart.** I know that both my husband and I want something better than we have. Making time for us is the difficult thing. My husband is a beautiful person and to the outside world we have a great marriage. What they don't see is the distraught person I am on the inside. I found a poem I wrote about fifteen years ago while throwing out old bits and pieces and the pain in that poem is the same pain as what I feel now, but now I know what it is I want and need, whereas back then I couldn't pinpoint it. Am I the teacher or do we learn together? At what point does one say enough is enough and I have to follow my own path? I feel like a very neglected female and I know this must change. I sincerely want this journey to be with my husband, I want to heal and energize him but there are times that I feel such immense pain in my heart just by being physically next to him. We have kissed passionately a few times recently and it was just so beautiful and

I do feel energy between us. I thank you for the work you do and for the insight.

Love, Rachel

Dear Rachel,

I am happy to hear that my book has been of value. **I was very touched by your words expressing your pain as a neglected woman – and I am sure they would speak directly to the hearts and beings of so many women. I feel it's important to say at the outset that the pain often experienced by women at the hands of man is usually not truly the 'fault' of man. In my view, the unhappy situation is the result of a collective absence of information and understanding.** As individuals we do not 'know' our bodies and their potential, let alone that of the opposite sex. Only a new perspective on sex can heal any rift that exists between us. Man and woman are self-contained units, and they are also designed to fit together as a single unit. However, it is difficult to sustain unity without a 'new' vision of sex.

I can definitely say that yes, for sure your husband is your man, and your partner for exploring love. Having worked with couples for almost 20 years now, I can say this with confidence. Many couples come to our workshops on the verge of separation, they hardly ever make love, and there is a great 'distance' between their hearts. But as soon as they begin to experiment with a new sexual approach, the connection is quickly re-established again. Many couples say that they experience the week as a 'second honeymoon'. It is so simple really, and what is required is a shift in perspective about sex. Plus you need a willingness to explore and experiment with sex. For men this can be more challenging as often men are quite identified with the conventional mode of sex and ejaculation; however, the rewards of changing these patterns are enormous and inestimable. If you can feel the spark in a kiss, then for sure that spark will be possible in all situations.

And yes, at times you can guide him by telling him how you feel, and share from the heart what feels right for your body. When you feel old pains rising in you, give them way, allow them to move out of you, do not repress them and do not try to understand them. Just let the tears flow and co-operate with your body. This is part of a deep cellular cleansing and purifying of your system. I also suggest that you meditate on your breasts for a half hour every day to support this healing process. As explained in the book, breasts are the positive energy awakening poles in a woman's body, and making them the focus of your awareness (also during sex) encourages feminine qualities.

It also helps to read to each other from the book, so you can hear the information together, without you having to tell him everything. Then decide on a few 'love keys' to experiment with and begin to make dates to make love. **Sex is something you do together, but at the same time it is an individual quest too. In this sense there is a lot you yourself can 'do' to change the atmosphere within and around you using your own awareness. By being more relaxed, receptive and feminine you can invite and create the quality of love that you are longing for.** There are no techniques involved – basically it is not what you do, but 'how' you do it. And that 'how ' is 'with awareness' - to be more conscious transforms the experience.

My tantra master Osho says, "Tantra is the transformation of sex into love through the awareness," which is so beautiful, it implies that awareness itself creates love. How simple and inspiring. And through my experience in teaching I see again and again how true this is. Couples who have been together for twenty, thirty, forty years are able to find each other in a fresh innocent way. As soon as you begin experimenting, I am sure you will find that you have the capacity to turn things around in your favor.

Love, Diana

8. Can tantric sex help me reconnect with my girlfriend?

Dear Diana,

I recently bought your book *The Heart of Tantric Sex*. I have just started it but I believe it is a great book so far. I bought the book, among many others, in order to explore and try to reconnect with my girlfriend. I am really interested in tantric sex. I want to ask you a couple questions nevertheless. Just to explain a little bit: I am 26 years old; I have been dating a girl for about a year. Some months ago, we started having sexual problems, as I had performance anxiety which started after we had a problem because I was feeling insecure since her previous relationship didn't seem to be completely over (although it was) but she still had some contact.

Our relationship involved some guilt as it started when she was still in that relationship, although her ex-boyfriend had already left the country for good. **Ever since the day I had performance anxiety and no erection, sex became something related to anxiety as opposed to pleasure – mostly for me – since every time I had performance anxiety and wouldn't reach an erection, it was the source of a fight and I felt terribly vulnerable at the time. (I guess mostly because of our 'wrong' beliefs that associate manliness with how good you are in bed.)** We don't have problems all the time about the occasions when I do lose an erection (although I believe sometimes they become silent arguments). Needless to say, this didn't only affect our sex life. It affected also our relationship as a whole (in my case I got so anxious that I wasted a lot of time just trying to 'fix' the problem so it affected my life). The emotions changed, things started to seem challenging; I guess I started seeing flaws where in the past I didn't. I started feeling perhaps less attracted, more reactive, etc. I have tried many things, but I like tantric sex because it involves learning how to relax around sex.

This is my case, and my question is: do you believe tantric sex could help me reconnect with her, and (mostly) with myself? At this point I have advanced in the reconnecting with myself step. I have learned many lessons from my relationship; I believe that it has also made me grow, but I still would like to reconnect more with my sexual energy (especially because I always felt so charged by it! Sex before this anxiety episode, almost in all my experiences and with previous partners, and of course with my current girlfriend, was really, really good). I tried some weeks ago just to have sex regardless of the results (erection or no erection) but I noticed that in spite of us doing that, which actually ended up in intercourse, we became less frequent. She also says it is because she feels less comfortable with her body since she gained some pounds in the last few months. And this is true, but I guess that it is a shallow perception to see things that way (although I guess both she and I do it), and also it's not all that bad because she still looks good! She is no supermodel and neither am I, but we are both normal looking I'd say, so I believe it shouldn't be an undermining situation for sex.

So I'd like to hear your words, maybe some tips on how to incorporate this new sex style in our lives. And one question about interpretation: in your book you talk about a guy who had two sexual partners and ends up with the one with whom he has more satisfying sex. **Now, does that mean according to the book that if sex is not satisfying you should look for a different partner (I don't believe so but just for clarification purposes), and if that's not the case, can tantric sex bring about good connection, energy or feelings between you and your partner?** Thank you so much.

Love, Antonio

Dear Antonio,

Since you wrote to me several weeks have passed, my apologies, so I am wondering how things are evolving with you and your girlfriend. To come to your last question first, the matter for clarification. Basically when sex is satisfying then couples are more likely to stay together. And discovering and learning the tantric style of sex can bring satisfaction, and be of great benefit to the relationship and its sustainability, as well as for your life in general. And this is because the awareness that is required for and during tantric sex generates love, respect, and togetherness. While in contrast, the more conventional mechanical orgasm focused style of sex does lead in many cases to some level of insensitivity, dissatisfaction, disconnection or separation.

I am sorry to hear that from a place of pleasure and confidence in sex you were unexpectedly confronted with performance issues. Certainly these erection issues have their root in the conventional style of sex, which is why it is so incredibly valuable to move out of that limited frame of sex. And discover a new definition of sex according to a tantric orientation. So yes, in answer to your basic question, I am convinced that tantric sex with your girlfriend will help your situation. And tantric sex will definitely bring about good feelings, connection and healing with any partner you have – now or in the future.

Naturally willingness is required on both sides, and at times unconscious reactions can come into play. So there has to be some awareness of the difference between emotions and feelings, and how to move forward in a creative way with these aspects of the personality/psychology. There are two chapters toward the end of *The Heart of Tantric Sex* that deal with this aspect and I would also recommend that you get hold of the book *Tantric Love – Feeling versus Emotion: Golden Rules to Make Love Easy* where the subject is elaborated and laid out very clearly.

You ask for some tips on how to incorporate this new sex style into your lives.

Basically you have to consciously create time and space for making love, and try out some of the guidelines/suggestions made in the book, so you can make a shift from theory into hands-on practice. In so doing you gradually learn how to become 'tantric' during the sexual exchange. It is a learning stays with you for life. The tantric way of being is not something you have to relearn for yourself each time with start with a new woman. You may of course have to introduce a woman to another way of being but that is another aspect. The basic aspect is that you, as an individual, transform on many levels.

And the younger you are when you do this turnaround, the easier.

So in this sense **things are looking good because at twenty-six your current sexual difficulties have pushed you to explore and find out more about sex. And that enquiry is the greatest blessing for your life, even though the actual impotence experiences have been emotionally challenging and confronting for you.**

The Heart of Tantric Sex lays out the 'love keys' and basic guidelines for practice, and it is then a matter of experimenting with them. Basically at the end of the day, it is not 'what' you do, but 'how' you do it. Tantric sex is definitely not a technique, or a set of rules; instead it is a new orientation that you grow and expand into. One of the first steps is to take the emphasis away from orgasm. This immediately reduces the performance aspect; you don't have to achieve anything. Even erection! There is also the suggestion on how to enter woman without erection - soft penetration. Making love frequently, talking with each other about your experiences, plus reading and then rereading the book will help you a lot. Through your personal practice slowly the level of understanding deepens, and there will be a change in your mind, and how you think about sex. And this is really what we are aiming for, a change in the mind, so that the reality of the body can be acknowledged and embraced for what it is. There is a book, Tantric Sex for Men, which you may find valuable. Included are many sharing's/reports from men during their tantric exploration that will interest, support, encourage and inspire you. I do hope this message answers most of your queries, and do write again if there is something I have overlooked.

Love, Diana

Dear Diana,

I have received your e-mail. With great satisfaction I have to say that it has answered many things. Also things have become better and better with time. As you said, this experience that has had a painful emotional side has also brought about a desire of searching for new frames of behavior, for new things and especially to know more about myself, and in this sense, that experience has been a blessing and a possibility of growth for me. I must say that I already bought those two books you recommended to me – nice coincidence – but I haven't got deeply into them yet. I consider that they could be valuable to my relationship. I talked to my girlfriend about tantric sex about a week ago, and how this approach to sex had started changing our sexual experience (for me and even with performance issues because I changed a lot the 'need-to-perform' approach in my mind). I'm not sure if it sounded a bit odd to her, but as you said, the most important thing is that it brings about change in me as an individual, and obviously this growth will also help and bring more love to our relationship.

One question that I still have (and that has been better recently since I believe I have been more loving lately to her), is why we humans see so much with our 'mind-eyes'? So much labeling with these eyes, so little room for love, and then it is a kind of love that depends on emotion and circumstance. I mean those eyes that tell us nice or ugly, fat or fit, naggy and unlovable and all those sort of labels of the things that can easily be noticed like physical appearance and behaviors... and then we create stories about these labels and love becomes even harder. I have been working on this, mainly by accepting every part of my whole 'self-construction' (or ego) and trying to transcend it, because I think that if you see with more loving eyes, the eyes that see more the essence of someone (like the soul), then you can give more love and also be more loving to yourself. This, I believe, is not an easy endeavor and that is why I ask you if tantric sex sees like that, like deep into someone else. **I think it is funny how our mind tricks us, because when love seems more present I see my girlfriend as really beautiful, and when the other labeling mind-eyes come into play I find myself labeling, comparing, not-accepting (especially not accepting of me and my behavior I'd say)... but I hope these all can be transcended.** I really appreciate your answer, Diana. I really like your books as you can see, since I already bought three of them! Have a great day, many blessings and love to your life,

Love, Antonio

Dear Antonio,

A quick mail in response to yours, for which thank you. I am pleased to hear that you are viewing your situation in a more positive light. A short comment on your observation: "Why we humans see so much with our 'mind-eyes', so much labeling with these eyes…" Yes, the superficiality in our society around the body and appearance is very sad for humanity. External transient aspects are given emphasis, while the inner eternal qualities are ignored and undervalued. Certainly in my experience the outside and how a person looks is no indicator of their sensitivity and inner beauty. So in this sense tantra offers a radical departure point, where one discovers and lives according to inner qualities and values, and especially around body/sex/attraction etc.

Through changing sexual approach one naturally aligns with higher spiritual vibrations that are transforming and the body becomes more beautiful with an inner beauty that shines through. I am sure everything will unfold in a wonderful way for you, and your intelligence, insights and curiosity will be great assets. Wish you the very best.

Love, Diana

9. It is clear for me that I must separate

Dear Diana,

Earlier this year I participated in your Making Love Retreat. I want to write you because many things have happened since and my partner and I have separated. On the second to last day I told him that I could no longer force my body to live the hard style of sex with him. He replied that this statement threatened his whole liveliness. Back then I did not see and recognize that this was absolutely true. Only with time I came to realize how little we were able to live and share together. He has had hardly any lively, joyful impulses since then, and I did not want to take responsibility for this part alone. During vacations this summer, for no apparent reason, he twice made very hurtful and disrespectful remarks to me during sex. I felt totally used and depreciated by him. Only after a while I came to the realization that he is not able to see me. Of course, this is due to his difficult childhood experiences and the hatred for his mother that he projects onto all women - and especially me, as his woman. **And also, my own childhood experiences with my father who ignored me and could only see himself.** He wanted to be alone and therefore drugged me with sleeping pills for many years. Screaming or showing any feelings were not allowed at all. I realized how much I was willing to let myself be used by 'man' hoping and keeping up the illusion that I may get attention and be given value through it. This very deep and old pattern is now allowed to heal and change. I meditate regularly, hold my breasts, the way you recommended me to do. And I hope in the right moment I will meet a man who is able to see and appreciate me when I also appreciate and honor myself. I send you cordial greetings. The seminar was far-reaching and very, very important for me. Thank you.

Love, Crystal

Dear Crystal,

Thank you for sharing with me about your changed situation. When a person is so clear in insight and intention, as you are, then it is very good to move forward without looking backwards. It seems to me that you have a realistic view of what is going on, and it is advisable to act responsibly and move on, as you have done. With this level of awareness you can create the environment for deep love to manifest in your life. With your kind of trust and clarity all good things, love and light are bound to follow.

It is nice that you enjoy doing the breast meditation and, as you have probably realized, this inner focus is a great support and nourishing resource for you day by day. Doing breast meditation will continue to transform your sexual energy as an individual, and in the absence of a partner. Also it will increase the 'inner sense' of you as a woman, and independent of man, which is very enriching.

Barry Long, one of my sources of inspiration, says that a woman should make love only where there is 'love enough'. So if you could feel that there was not enough love, honor, respect or willingness to be more conscious, then you have made the correct decision. **What I appreciate about your message is that you do not appear to be in an emotional state, where you are blaming your partner etc. You are talking about yourself more than him, which is a sign of clarity and integrity. Moving through in your courageous positive way, without drama and recrimination, will serve to strengthen your self-love, and thereby your love for all other beings.** May your life be infused with the joy of love each moment.

Love, Diana

10. After some time of marriage, sex got unbearable

Dear Diana,

I just started reading *Tantric Orgasm for Women* in Spanish, and I have so many doubts I would like to ask you about. Your book has really inspired my and given me some light in my reduced knowledge of sexuality and making love. Even though it has given me a completely different concept of making love, I still cannot reach the beautiful things you talk about.

I would like to tell you a little bit of my sexual history, so maybe that way you can understand. I'm thirty years old, and I've been married for three and a half years, and I have a one year old baby girl. My husband is a wonderful man, we got to know each other when I was twenty-four, and with almost no experience I starting 'making love' with him in the ordinary conventional way. I always enjoyed kissing and stimulating the clitoris but I've never been able to enjoy penetration. When we were dating it was just okay (I did it more to please him); but after some time, when we were married, it got unbearable, it even caused me to feel anger and frustration.

So I got into psychotherapy focused on the body, acupuncture, transpersonal therapy, meditations etc., and it has been getting better but still sex is not as pleasant as it is supposed to be. I was just with a good psychic and she told me that my first chakra was completely closed and that I was sexually abused at the age of five. I honestly don't remember anything so maybe it happened, and maybe it did not. I've been trying with my husband some of the ways you propose in the book but it is hard for him to stay with the erection without moving. I like it a lot more that way, but for him it is frustrating to lose the erection.

Please tell me what I can do. I don't want to give up on my pleasure, but I don't know what else to do. Can you give me any homework? Thank you very much for giving me some of your time and attention.

Love, Lara

Dear Lara,

It is delicate to answer your questions because there are so many aspects to them, so I will answer generally. Yes, the softer style of sex will help to heal and overcome the difficulties of the past, but it will need the co-operation, compassion, understanding and patience of your husband. He will need to find the willingness to be more slow and conscious, which includes losing his erection in certain situations. Probably most men, if not all, carry a very deeply rooted fear of impotence, so when erection is lost during sex these fears are touched. Usually men override this fear by increasing stimulation and excitement, but if a man is able to accept and relax into being non-erect, which is after all a natural state of the penis, the experience is an empowerment. He will feel himself more confident, grounded in his body, more manly.

Often unexpressed feelings will underlie the fear of losing

73

an erection, and it is very healing for a man to get in touch with these aspects, and to give way to any feelings that come to the surface. It could be tears, shivering or shaking, deep feelings of insecurity, helplessness or anything. Sometimes a man will cry from the deep relief experienced through not *having to have* an erection. The tension and performance pressures that man is burdened with in sex are able to dissolve and this will make a man's basic life/sexual energy stronger. Being able to reach to these levels of inner reality will in the long-term actually make a man become more 'potent' and establish a true 'male authority' in man.

It is also necessary for man (and woman) to realize that the female body opens up more slowly and needs more time than male body to be ready for sex. Often a woman's lack of pleasure and interest in sex is because her body is usually not truly open and prepared for man's entry. For accessing a deeper level of woman's sexual energy there needs to be a shift from the clitoris to the breasts. Her vagina is more secondary but then after a while a response or awakening is felt on a much deeper level in the vagina. When the vagina is more open and receptive then you will find it much easier to let man enter you, and you yourself will experience much greater pleasure.

Many women do observe that clitoral stimulation somehow 'disturbs' the vaginal environment, it feels hungry and excited, and this reduces the 'power' and 'purity' of the penetration as happens when the vagina is more relaxed and receptive. That is the basic reason why it is better to avoid clitoral stimulation as the starting point in sex. With stimulation of the clitoris you end up going along the excitement track of sex and building up to a climax, and not along the sensitivity track and being more relaxed in the here and now. On the surface it looks like the approach is just a denial of pleasure and orgasm and so on, but it's not. It is more about honoring the intelligence of our bodies and that will involve changing our minds about sex and rearranging how we go about it.

Regarding a psychic saying that you have some sexual abuse in your childhood. Sadly, we do live in a world where sexual abuse of innocent children is extremely common, so there is a possibility that something happened to you during your childhood.

Sometimes boundaries are crossed in subtle ways, but they are no less invasive. As a pretty young girl even the sexual vibrations coming from the 'look' in the eyes of a man, can be enough of a crossing of boundaries to cause bodily contraction and inner tension. Often a person will have some inkling that something went on, and I have heard therapists say that if there is any hint of a memory from childhood, then in all probability it is true. In your case you cannot remember anything, and no memory has come to the surface during your different therapies. In a way it is not important to find out if abuse happened or not because the way to heal these tensions is the same for us all no matter the source – and that is through conscious slow loving sex.

The main thing to do now is to begin making love more often in the spirit of exploration, allowing whatever happens, erection or no erection. Be open to whatever feelings wish to move through you. Allowing tears etc., as already mentioned earlier in relation to your husband, is healing and purifying, so it is beautiful if you can be open to yourselves, and open to each other. Be simple and do not have great expectations that everything should be perfect right away. When your expectations are not met, you will naturally feel disappointed, and this will distract you and take your energy and attention. It also means you will fail to see anything positive that may be happening on other levels or in different ways. Healing and balancing takes time, so just be willing to take small steps. It will be very helpful if you read my book together so you both gain a mutual and common understanding of what you are doing, and why you are doing it.

Best wishes to you and your husband.

Love, Diana

Dear Diana,

I really want to thank you for giving me your attention. **I've been talking with my husband about going to one of your courses next year and he's being thinking about it, but he is afraid of**

being exposed. He wants me to ask you if the sexual exercises are done with everybody there watching. He is a wonderful man, who has taught me wonderful things about life, but he is very square in the mind (through his education and job) and he definitely has made a great effort to open up to my unprovable world, to the things he cannot see. I hope you understand what I mean. I'm doing all that I can to be there next year because I think it will be a great opportunity for both, but I need to explain to him, and I need to know if this is not too eccentric for him. I would really appreciate if you could clarify a little bit on this aspect.

Love, Lara

Dear Lara,

Please assure your husband that the course is very professional and respectful of the individual and of the couple, and we seek to make the experience as relaxing and unthreatening as possible. We create a very safe and intimate environment. There is absolutely no exposure of any kind, and all lovemaking happens in the privacy of the bedroom. **We talk about making love in a very open and straightforward way, but all practice takes place in privacy. There are no group structures that involve other participants, all the 'work' happens exclusively within the couple.**

If you do not wish to talk to any other couple during the retreat, then this is also okay. We try to reduce the amount of social chitchat that happens so easily when people get together, so that couples can be free to be with themselves and without having to interact with others.

I also wish to say that coming to a course is not absolutely essential in order to learn a new way of making love. My books are complete in the sense that they are written for people I imagined I would never meet in a live teaching situation. So if you cannot make it to a workshop, you can still do the exploration. The workshop simply acts as a jump-start, giving fresh input and the possibility of some practice.

But the real 'work' starts when you get home and back into the routine of daily life. Here the challenge is to make the time for you both. I suggest that you don't postpone. Find a babysitter for your child and arrange for you and your husband to have scheduled time together. Without doubt your child will also benefit tremendously from the loving vibrations that you and your husband will begin to emanate.

Love, Diana

11. She's the woman I want to love and cherish with all my being

Dear Diana,

We are still astonished at how much the week with you is changing our vision, perception, feeling, and being. As individuals, and us together as a couple. Even if my commitment to my woman was absolutely clear on a deep level beforehand, it has become even more clear that she is the woman I want to love and cherish with all my being.

If before I knew and felt that hot sex was not an end in itself, rather a drug like others (drinking, smoking, working, thinking), what you're saying and radiating has made really tangible what I felt deep inside me ever since I can remember. Spirituality, connection, just simple ordinary nature, freed from concepts and fears. It really is reassuring. Both of us are feeling a deep proximity and we both enjoy being in each other's presence.

For me personally, the past two weeks since the group with you have been rich in feelings and learning. I have felt very vulnerable, under self-attack and feeling little self-esteem. My ego has been trying to make sense of this life and wondering what am 'I' on this planet for, what am 'I' good for, and who is this 'I' anyway? There was an enormous feeling of loss at the end of the group because obviously the very close all day contact with my partner could not continue the same way in daily life. By today, however, 'I' is much more back in the body and in the here and now, and some other fragments of ego have probably fallen off.

I notice I have less fear of the future, less need to be somebody to survive, I feel more be and let live, and sense much more contact with my partner even over the distance when we are apart. It feels like letting love flower into spring!

Love, Manfred

Dear Manfred,

It has been a joy to receive your heart-warming message that reveals the beauty and love within you. Thank you both for your intelligence, clarity and sensitivity. And it is touching to hear that you recognize how bits of your personality and ego are dropping off to reveal the real loving you. Good that you can watch the fascinating process from a distance, it certainly reflects of the depth of your enquiry. It was a real pleasure to share the week with you, and to now be on the same journey to the simple here and now.

Love, Diana

12. My girlfriend is afraid of trying a new way of making love

Dear Diana,

As you know I have separated from my girlfriend, a couple of years after participating in the Making Love Retreat. She fell in love with another man, and the sudden break up with her was quite hard in the beginning. But I feel that I was able to let go quite quickly. Maybe the spiritual orientation I have learned with you has helped me to accept life, to live the moment, and to realize that everything is impermanent.

The bigger challenge for me now is that my new girlfriend is very afraid of trying this new way of making love. She likes your book but she is not yet ready to let go of the common way of having sex. Do you have experience with such a situation and how I can I deal with it? For now I'm being patient and trying not to force her. Thanks in advance for your words.

Love, Patrick

Dear Patrick,

It is good to hear that you were able to let go of your girlfriend with relative ease and understanding. And of course I am very pleased to know that you have met another woman. I suggest you start out with yourself first, and see what you can do, from your side, to influence and elevate the experience. Be more sensitive, more present, keep excitement at a low level, and be 'cool'.

I know it's quite a challenge when a woman wants to go for the usual orgasm, but the less you can be involved or get caught up in it yourself, the better. Be there for her, but do not partake of it. If you can avoid ejaculation in these circumstances then that is a great step, in the sense that you do not discharge your own energy and vitality. But if it is not possible to avoid ejaculation then that is perfectly under-standable too. **Often the excitement that a woman builds up in order to reach a peak will cause a man to ejaculate; there is usually very little he can do about it.**

Of course coming to a workshop with us is optimum, but at the same time not essential. To encourage her you can always say that she can go back to what she was doing before, if she wishes. In any event, what we teach is not a black or white situation, this or that. Starting out always and only implies bringing more awareness into whatever you are doing, more awareness to what is present and that very awareness will be transforming. Woman basically appreciates and values when a man is present to her, so if you can develop this quality and side of yourself, then she will in all likelihood slowly open up to other possi-bilities.

Love, Diana

Dear Diana,

It is many months since I last wrote to you, and I took your words to heart, but here I am again and I hope that is okay that I ask you something again. I'm still together with my new girlfriend but awareness in sex is quite difficult with her. Sometimes we have a nice experience with no orgasm, but most of the time she can't deal with this kind of making love and wants to go the usual way. And she says she doesn't want to attend the course. I'm quite patient but I would like to develop making love. What can I do? Is it a reason to leave a relationship? My therapist says it is not a good reason to leave. So at the moment the higher knowledge I received during your course makes it more complicated to live a relationship. On the other hand I would love to live it.

Love, Patrick

Dear Patrick,

I am sorry to hear that having the knowledge you received during the course is making your new relationship difficult to sustain. At the same time it is so valuable to have another view of sex, especially since you are a young man. It is a shame that your girlfriend is not so interested in trying out new ways. This can easily happen because the sexual conditioning is deep and we become identified with how we have sex; it is part of who we think we are. To begin to change the way we make love does require the willingness to take a little distance, with a more enquiring mind. As I said in my previous letter to you, the best you can do in the situation is to remain in the awareness, remembering the key is not what you do but how you do it.

Sometimes people get the idea that tantric sex has to happen only in stillness and without movement. But this is not true. Stillness is only one option. There can be movements that have no goal or direction, movements that are infused with presence and inner stillness. So perhaps you yourself have made up some ideal of how it should look like. If she does like orgasm, then you can encourage her to postpone it and also suggest that she relax into it as she builds up to a climax. Usually the body gets tense as it does this but the very tension itself restricts the expansion of energy. So there are subtle things that can be 'done' by being aware, even in the conventional way.

It is not easy for you, I am sure, to have a longing and the information to elevate the sexual experience. At the same time the patience you are practicing is a very good quality to develop. I do feel that sometimes this longing for higher experiences can be a reason to leave a relationship; it really depends on the individual. In my early thirties I left a relationship so that I could find a man who was interested in exploring sex on a deeper level.

Instead of thinking about whether you should leave her or not, another way perhaps, is to begin manifesting a woman who is like-minded and like-spirited as you are. You can do this by connecting with your solar plexus, where the source of longing is usually located, and from this place begin to radiate light and love. So you are not thinking with your mind or you are not fantasizing about an ideal person, but radiating an inner longing outward into the world and thereby inviting and drawing the 'right' person to you. Enjoy your explorations!

Love, Diana

Dear Diana,

Thank you so much for your quick and very helpful reply. I will put your suggestions into action. Yes, I do have a bit of an idea that stillness is the way, but that is because I like it so much! At least we do this sometimes, and for that I am grateful. I feel more relaxed about the situation now, especially when I realize that I do not have to decide something about the relationship, but just wait and see what life offers me.

Love, Patrick

13. My wife has lost interest in sex since birth of our son

Dear Diana,

A few days ago I went to a family-counseling center in Germany again. I wanted to get advice regarding the missing and dysfunctional physical contact to my wife – something I miss very much.

The psychologist recommended to me that I attend one of your seminars, but I do not know yet whether my wife is willing to participate in a couple retreat at all. Neither do I know whether this program is suitable for us. We are both in our early fifties. We have a son who will turn eleven this year. Since the birth of our son my wife says that she has no longing for sex anymore – probably because of the hormones. Many years ago we already had a sexual relationship, separated, and then twelve years ago we came back together again.

I think the aspect of sexual lust was too important to me in the beginning of our marriage. When the child was born and one year later my wife still did not show any sign of tenderness and talking about it was impossible, I started to go crazy inside. I felt hopelessly trapped. The only possibilities I saw were staying or leaving and I did not want to give up everything and hoped for improvement.

Now I feel I am ready to search my path. I also still hope a little bit that my wife could also thaw. She grew up in a family where physical touch was very much avoided. They even avoided shaking hands. My question is: What possibilities can you offer us? Do you recommend us to take part in a course? I would be very happy to know if your program is suitable for us.

Love, Ken

Dear Ken,

Thank you for writing to me about your situation with your wife, and I find it touching that you are again and again looking for new ways to reach her, without giving up. Many couples do come to our groups with this same sense of great physical distance but usually after one week of guidance and some practice in lovemaking the difficulties fall away easily.

A woman's loss of interest in sex after birth is quite common. A woman is likely to feel much more sensitive and the hot more aggressive style of sex is not so attractive to her

because it does not suit her body. I feel if you approach her in a soft way, as suggested in our books and courses, then she will be more open to your attentions. I know many women who managed sex quite soon after birth when it was in the conscious and softer style.

In truth the problem between you and your wife is not 'personal', as in you and her, as it seems on the surface. The gap is there because of no concrete information about sex and male/female energies working together. I am sure that if you talk to your wife about your feelings, your longings, the book, the course, your wish to change something, she is sure to respond to your love and sincerity.

I am confident that you and your wife will benefit from participation, as individuals and as a couple. At the same time because of the delay until you can participate you can start reading the book to give you an orientation. Perhaps you can even begin to try out some of the suggestions given in the book. Start with simple things like eye contact, or breathing together.

All the best to you in your search for more love in your life.

Love, Diana

Dear Diana,

Thank you for your kind letter. I leave today for a few days of vacation and would like to talk there to my wife about the possibility of making love in a new way.

I have the book *The Heart of Tantric Sex* and have read some of it already. Some things I try to practice too, like being more connected to my body and staying in the moment. My wife behaves sometimes more like a man. She reacted with a verbal attack when she saw the book! So I hope that it goes well and I send you greetings.

Love, Ken

Dear Ken,

It is perfect that you have a vacation now so that you can give some time to being together. Yes, sometimes women do react in a more hard and 'male' way but this is just an outcome of the sexual misunder-standing and conditioning. Underneath women are usually as soft as butter (out of the fridge!) and as sweet as honey. Try to melt her down with your love and presence without putting pressure on her. Remember that woman's body takes longer than man's to be fully open, and the breasts are the way into her energy system. So be sure to grant her the time to relax into herself. Naturally because you have not had sex for some time you will want to go the whole way immediately, but I advise you to take it slowly and not to have great expectations. You will need to be patient and willing to take small steps at a time. Best wishes to you.

Love, Diana

14. I do not feel like being intimate with my husband

Dear Diana,

I am writing to you at the recommendation of my therapist. During the session last Wednesday I expressed to her my great concern at the moment about planning to participate in the Making Love Retreat with my husband because right now I do not feel like being close to him at all – either in intimacy or in general daily life.

The most concerning point is that I do not feel like being naked next to him. And I do not wish to see him naked. I feel an immense aliveness in my body and sexual organs since a few weeks when the Pandora Box was opened.

This opening corresponded to the awareness that my sexual life was not satisfying enough in pleasing my partner, avoiding my real needs and desires as well as avoiding the painful subject with him. It also meant I felt a very sudden and strong aliveness of my sexual energy which gave me no choice but to address the subject with myself, and with my husband. But I do not feel like sharing all this energy with him.

I would like to be able to read what you have to say about

these points as I am aware that it might be 'a problem' to participate in the retreat with those feelings. Maybe it won't be a problem but I'd prefer to clarify it before going any further in any possible bookings. My husband is not feeling the way I feel, he is comfortable with a 'whatever situation'.

Love, Victoria

Dear Victoria,

It happens quite often that couples come to our retreat in a state of separation on some level. However, the reorientation you will be given very soon brings back to life the love and closeness. Of course there is no guarantee that this will happen, but our experience is that it does!

If for whatever reason this does not happen, then at the very least you will have received a lesson in life, and one that can then be used as a basis for further relationships. So in this sense what we teach is beyond the couple, and for the individual. Also with a new orientation on emotions and feelings, if perhaps separation does ever take place, it is more likely to happen in a loving, caring way and not in a destructive, emotional way. **At present, if you decide to separate, there is every chance that the same pattern comes into play with the next man sooner or later.** Hope these few words help you in getting clear about your next step.

Love, Diana

Dear Diana,

Thank you for your words. They really answered the questions I had in mind and even gave me more perspective on the possible outcomes if we participate in the retreat. It is very soothing right now for me to have your feedback; I am getting some rest and able to slow down the 'thinking' and surrender more to what 'is'. I deeply appreciate your support.

Love, Victoria

15. Our personal discoveries based on your books

Dear Diana,

My main interest in writing is to join you in your efforts to help lovers discover the new dimension that we can reach if we just let go and change our reactionary and compulsive approach to sex. **Your book has corroborated some of the findings my partner and I discovered recently.** What's most amazing is that your teachings came to us at just the right time and helped us by giving meaning and putting in perspective this natural and organic way to loving that we have been experiencing. The timeliness and synchronicity of this discovery (your teachings) remains a mystery to both of us. Indeed someone once said that the book and the woman (or man) that will change the course our lives would find us without our looking for them.

There were certain aspects of our relationship that we had found needed to be realigned. We have been and are now in the process of doing just that.

I've listed below some of my reflections based on having read your books, as well as our independent empirical findings.

- That which is the most sacred activity, sex, has been turned into the most profane. What's supposed to liberate us from our egoic consciousness' programming has become one of its most powerful and addictive 'routines' (borrowing the term from cybernetics). It's like we are so fixated in form that we've become oblivious to its complimentary aspect, emptiness. Therefore, the term 'spiritual sex' may seem an oxymoron to many, yet we can't be truly whole unless we integrate both, body and spirit. The fact that you make this amply clear in your books certainly makes a difference... a BIG difference... between your message and that of others.
- Perhaps the reason we (men) are driven to give woman as many orgasms as we can get them to elicit has its roots in

the ego's need to reinforce itself (as a great lover). Our real motivation is oftentimes disguised as an altruistic act. Appeasing the ego can be more powerful in its effects than the most wonderful orgasm, and far more addictive. Arguably, this is one of the main components of goal-driven sex. You mention this in your book but it can't be overemphasized. We've both realized that lovemaking has more to do with being than doing, more with flowing than attaining.

• We realized that orgasm is not the goal (this is in spite of the fact that neither of us had any problem reaching them and continue to enjoy them immensely when they happen). Lovemaking should not be goal-oriented. In actual fact, when we are joined in love, as suggested in your book, the movement of our bodies seems to be in response to the flow of energy that's taken place and not driven by our minds. We simply allow ourselves to respond by disengaging our rational minds from the act (letting go of all thoughts, images, etc.) Instead, we let our Self emerge and merge, manifesting itself through our body mind. Simply put, in true lovemaking there are no 'doers'. I guess we could call it 'authentic lovemaking' (as opposed to ersatz sex), although the term is somewhat of a misnomer given the action denoted by the verb.

• When we relax and the uncontrolled drive for pleasure and excitement ceases, it becomes possible to perceive the flow of energy as it deepens and intensifies. The sensation and response resulting from this exchange is very different from that produced by friction or activation of the body's erogenous zones. What is most interesting is that it (the energy) can't be controlled; quite the contrary, the more we let go the more it flows and intensifies.

• Given the relaxed nature of this exchange, lovemaking can go on for an indefinite amount of time. We came to realize that in reality we do not make love, but that love is simply allowed to happen, to be, in and through us. It's truly a meditative experience like no other.

- It became clear to me that I needed to develop my listening skills in order to effectively translate my partner's messages. I think the difficulty lies in the way we have been programmed, which causes us (men) to assume certain things and, on the basis of those assumptions, react, instead of responding according to what our partner really needs or wants. For example, it took me some time to process the fact that in order to get her to open up I needed to activate her breasts. This in spite of the fact that she had told me her clitoris would not respond, no matter how much stimulation it received, unless and until the energy began to flow from her upper body and breasts. In the same manner, I kept getting new toys to experiment with, although she had made it clear that the best 'toy' was my penis.

In order to open ourselves to this experience, we found it beneficial to prepare and predispose ourselves for it. The necessary sensitivity, as well as the sensibility, both sensory and emotional has to be there for the pathways to open. Also, our mental attitude has to be in synch. For instance, someone who relies on fantasy or mental images would have a very difficult time achieving this state since disengaging the mind, not engaging, is necessary. The same applies for someone who can only respond to high excitation /stimuli, such as those produced by a vibrator. For someone like that it would be very hard to perceive the energy flow and much less enjoy this form of lovemaking. It's likely that they would simply dismiss it altogether as rubbish.

I apologize for having written such a lengthy e-mail but have done so open-heartedly hoping that in a small way we may contribute to your research on the subject.

In closing, I would like to do so quoting T.S. Eliot since his words seem to have been written for all those who search for Love and are therefore most appropriate to the subject at hand.

We shall not cease from our exploration
And at the end of all our exploring
Will be to arrive where we started
And know the place for the first time.

May the Light of your True Self be your guide always.

Love, Rafael

Chapter 3

Emotional Aspects

1. I have the impression that I am constantly emotional
2. Positive resources lying in past that do not classify as emotions
3. A load of feelings and emotions
4. Becoming aware of my low-grade emotions
5. Noticing negative after-effects of ejaculation
6. Experiencing that my fear is healed by love
7. I get closed because I think my partner doesn't love me
8. I am desperate and I question my whole being as a man
9. Sex is difficult for me because of high expectations and baby wish
10. Experiencing deep sadness and lethargy
11. Feeling more often frustration and boredom
12. I really have no clue how to deal with my 'blocks'
13. These old emotions are somehow 'sitting' on my sexuality
14. Our journey with love and letting go of emotions

The chapter on emotional aspects deals with a domain where a great lack of clarity and insight exists, and is based on the understanding that there is a fundamental difference between 'emotions' and 'feelings'. Emotions are in fact an accumulation of unexpressed feelings from the past. If and when the level of accumulated emotion is high it easily leads to difficulties in sex and/or problems in relationship, in the present. So in this way what happened in the past, and what is actually happening in the present, get confused. Emotions tend to temporarily obscure the love present between two people, and 'emotionality' will display itself in complaining, blaming, arguing and power/ego struggles.

Love is then experienced as something with good times and bad times, the proverbial 'ups and downs'. How to separate authentic feelings from destructive emotions, as well as how to deal with these emotions, is described in detail in the book *Tantric Love – Feeling versus Emotion: Golden Rules to Make Love Easy.*

1. I have the impression that I am constantly emotional

Dear Diana,

Regarding making love: I have the impression that I am 'constantly emotional'. To create free space for myself I stopped everything for now in order to find a way back to myself, first of all. I have been doing Yoga, Feldenkrais and learning Spanish. My partner and I work together and I look for relaxation and balance because I have too much work, and what impressed me most was when you said that teaching the seminar was fun for you both and not work. For us working in the company is a fight for survival every day. We have a plumbing business and currently we have several employees. This is pure stress: either we have too much or too little work. After the second time of spending a week with you I have the feeling that I come into contact with very deep, old patterns of beliefs. I have already done so much bodywork and until now I have not managed to bring the deep realizations into my life. As if I silently knew all along that there is another truth, and another possibility whereby to live. It got very interesting for me when my partner started to get involved. And started to let go of his 'orgasm fixation'. Since then I have been floundering. Without orientation, a fear of losing control – who am I, and what is my value as a woman when he is not immediately senseless with excitement? Very stupid. Therefore, **I have to feel into myself - which is not so easy at all, especially when I realize how little I can actually feel and how much I was focused and concen-**

trated on what was going on with my partner. **I can feel myself almost only through pain.** This is why I love the Five Tibetan exercises, because afterward I can feel all my muscles. I think I can work more on this.

One thing that also is obvious to me with regard to emotionality is that I have the impression that I am in a state of shock. In a freeze in which I cannot move. I have the feeling that I cannot go on at all. If I move, I move like a robot. If I manage to really move my body it is good. I, for example, recently did a dance meditation in the night for the first time. Last night I could not manage and I woke up stiff. Is there a trick, a tip of how to overcome this point more easily? Everything in my body resists and cries for no movement. It cries I do not want, no change! In this cesspool I at least know where I am. I cannot yet distinguish between when I am really exhausted and it is better to rest, and when movement is indicated.

Love, Karen

Dear Karen,

Thank you for writing. Yes, sometimes the emotional state can feel like being in a freeze or in a shock. And it is this that makes it *so* hard to get moving. There is no real easy way to overcome it, except to 'force' yourself because you love yourself! If you don't manage, then *at least* you know why you are feeling bad; it is no longer a mystery. This distance in itself is going to make you feel better. Not fully, but a bit.

Sometimes the fight against doing something positive for yourself can be on a deeper level a resistance to the present. You keep things simple; you just do anything like shaking, jumping up and down, or gibberish, and find ways to release the tension. There is a problem with using your level of exhaustion as a monitor for what to do next, because emotion itself will make a person feel exhausted. If you really do feel that you are genuinely exhausted (and lack of sleep can definitely be a source of emotions) then go to bed early, sleep well, and see how you feel in the morning. If you wake and do not feel 'refreshed' in any way, or more 'positive' in your outlook, then that is telling you that you will need to get moving the next day. Best wishes to you.

Love, Diana

2. Positive resources lying in past that do not classify as emotions

Dear Diana,

I participated with my wife in the Making Love Retreat recently. Afterwards I had the following thoughts about your talk on knowing the difference between emotions and feelings: Emotions derive from old hurts, patterns etc. – and affect my relationship to myself and to my partner in a negative way. You described the situation perfectly. This means the old feelings are 'stored' in us. You also gave the example of a child that again and again has to struggle for the love of its parents by being very good or trying hard – sometimes even in vain.

Feelings happen/arise in the present and when they are expressed they affect the relationship to myself and to my partner in a positive way.

In this model, however, I missed a third dimension: the positive 'old feelings' (or emotions?) that derive from the past and can be activated in us again and again. We can use them as resources. They belong to the past, are stored in our bodies and minds but as emotions (?) and affect relationships/life in a positive way.

I am talking about my own experience: my mother's fear of losing my father was present from the moment I was born because he had to leave for Russia one day prior to my birth. Of course I also felt my mother's fear to lose us children. At the same time, however, I also felt her unconditional love that I can feel until today and that is a good basis for me to 'trust the world'. Then I was also allowed to feel my grandfather's unconditional love. We lived with him until my father came back.

Then there were also many moments of joy and acknowledgement in my childhood, youth, and adult life and it helps me to remember my past.

In her book *Joy, Inspiration and Hope*, Verena Kast suggests to write a biography of joy. I think it is very helpful to let these positive energies reverberate in me – also for my ability to love (myself and others). And maybe we should focus more on these positive experiences and emotions/feelings of the inner child in general? I am wondering: Would you rather call them emotions or feelings – or do we need a third term? Thank you for the various impulses and the beautiful inner experiences that we received in your seminar!

Love, Konrad

Dear Konrad,

I appreciate your writing to me with your observations/insights into this important subject. Yes, you are absolutely right, there are definitely experiences that lie in the past that classify as positive resources, and not as emotions. And for most of us certainly not everything that lies in the past was negative. But for many people who have had strong negative influences in their early years, the tendency is that the negative is remembered, it holds the power, not the positive. It is a gift for your life that the positive has played such a significant part in your formation. Being able to feel and experience the unconditional love of your mother and your grandfather is a tremendous resource and will have helped you to becoming the loving person that you are.

Thank you for raising this aspect of positive resources lying in the past - a reminder to honor their significance. It certainly has been true for me in the sense that I had my first tantric or 'blissful' experience when I was only seven years old. And to this day I can feel it as a source of light and love inside me that I can hook up with any time I turn inwards. So you are right to emphasize that it is very helpful to let these positive energies consciously reverberate within. It would be very nice for everyone to be more focused on how the positive in the past is supporting us. However, unfortunately it is the negative/unresolved issues from the past that are more easily motivated/triggered – hence the destructive pattern in relationships, and hence my focus on ways to deal with these disturbances.

I often hesitate to use the term 'inner child' because sometimes, from my perspective, emotions are passed off/indulged as aspects of the 'inner child', when that is not necessarily so. Instead I often see an 'emotional' inner child. I feel that the quality you want to preserve, bring to the foreground and nourish can perhaps better be described as the 'innocent child'. Again, many thanks for your input on this aspect.

Love, Diana

3. A load of feelings and emotions

Dear Diana,

We participated in your Making Love Retreat and we enjoyed the time very much. Our sexual journey continues to develop and gives us new experiences again and again. A wide, loving landscape surrounds us. I am very happy about it.

The reason I write you, however, is because of a load of feelings and emotions!

We both have children and we live in relatively distant places. I am a single mother and he shares his task with the mother of his daughter. We are bound to our living places and we do not have much time left to be together. For me these circumstances again and again trigger crises and now again I find myself in the midst of one. With your help I am beginning a journey. I think that by now I am able to separate feelings and emotions. My emotions bring to light the issues of 'not having space', 'not being loved and accepted'. Deep wounds from the past. I know this. It is wonderful how love begins to grow anew since I have started to dedicate time to keeping an eye on emotions and feelings. Many smaller gateways have opened and I see connections. I have just started this journey, but I feel very clearly that this is good for me.

There is one issue, however, that confuses me: I really want to spend time with my partner. I want to have (more) time together for projects, to talk, to make love, to help each other and to share everyday life. As I understand my partner, he seems to give priority to other things. For him, first of all his daughter and the relationship to his family are important. He is much more able to live in the moment. I experienced that these circumstances stir my emotions. But they are also needs. Am I to let them go like my emotions? Even though I feel a lot of love for my partner, a feeling of unhappiness and of sadness remains. What do you think about it? I would be happy to hear from you.

Love, Astrid

Dear Astrid,

From what you say, it sounds like you are managing with your situation as best possible and having some very interesting insights. It is a challenge when there are children/families from other relationships, and as I see it there is little that you can do about the situation except to accept it how it is. When things are deeply accepted the tension falls away and you will feel yourself much more relaxed in the moment. And you are right; sometimes emotions do come from not having needs fulfilled. Sometimes the needs can be 'mind' needs/ideas rather than essential needs.

For instance, it is less usual for a couple to live apart, so the mind will convince you that ultimately it is better to live together. It becomes a need, and one in your case that is not being fulfilled and a cause for unhappiness. Couples who live together often find themselves living very parallel rather than truly 'together'. Often they will take each other for granted and give their partnership less value and therefore make less time for each other. When you see each other *less* frequently you are *definitely* more present and alive to each other. So it is helpful if you recognize that there are positive aspects to your situation.

To fill in the gap you will need to find ways to nourish yourself, create more personal time and enjoy being with your own body. Do some exercises, dance, and meditate on the breasts etc., or read Barry Long or Osho, so that you feel inwardly nourished even if your partner is not with you as often as you would like him to be. I remember you both well, a beautiful and loving couple. Best wishes to both of you.

Love, Diana

Dear Diana,

Loving thanks for your answer, very nice to hear from you. Many things have moved and become clear since. These are wonderful experiences that I am able to make – also when the recognizing of my emotions keeps me on my toes. I will be really fit when things continue like this!

Love, Astrid

4. Becoming aware of my low-grade emotions

Dear Diana,

The very special week with you both is still vibrating in us – thank you again so much! Last week the emotions hindered us at times to practice making love, but now we are really eager to do so, and have already done so! I want to write something about becoming aware of my low-grade emotions.

When I heard your talk on how to distinguish between emotions and feelings for the first time, I didn't feel really that I was being an emotional person in my everyday life because I fight with my husband only very rarely. Now, one year later, after hearing the talk for the second time I find myself being extremely emotional, on a more subtle level, but somehow permanently, and especially towards my husband. This became clear to me when I heard your term 'low-grade emotional'.

Being conditioned and raised in a quite controlled manner (by my parents and other adults who praised me for being so 'well-balanced') I always tried to avoid conflict with my partner. In case of argument or conflict I would immediately withdraw back internally; it often felt like 'freezing'. So when an emotion was released inside of me, instead of expressing it (e.g. in fighting or blaming) I used to push it back at the same time and therefore 'recycled' it in a way. These recycled emotions built up over the years into an almost invincible wall between us, hindering in the end any loving feelings of any kind.

Now opening up towards myself, and my partner, I recently feel myself being a lot more 'high-grade' emotional, as only *now* **I learn to perceive and allow emotions within myself. This is often frightening to me. At the same time, it can be rewarding, when I manage to identify it** as just being an emotion – what a relief! I send a ray of light to you.

Love, Jasmin

Dear Jasmin,

So many thanks for your interesting message, and yes, it is a really positive step that you have noticed your low-grade emotions; congratulations on your insight, it is life changing. And yes, it is the way to go, to become high-grade emotional as part of the process of change, and to become more aware of when exactly the emotions are triggered within you. And then to 'work' on them (through movement etc., or releasing the old pains in tears for example as suggested in my books) so that you can access and melt down all that has become frozen within you. **It does take courage to confront the emotional state, but as you have experienced, it's a big relief! And how quickly everything gets simplified.** I hope that the good feelings created between you during the week together are growing and flowing beautifully, and wish you both a loving summer.

Love, Diana

5. Noticing negative after-effects of ejaculation

Dear Diana,

It is unbelievable how much has changed in the past months since the Making Love Retreat. When I think about what has happened to me, tears are running and I am infinitely grateful for these experiences and for this gift in my life. Again and again, I am confused and I keep thinking: "This can't be true. I am for sure on some sort of trip." But the trip does not seem to end. It looks as if, for the very first time in my life, I realize that I have treated my body badly and that I can stop this without effort from one moment to the other. The physical symptoms that come up are so strong, that the beautiful sensation of having an orgasm is nothing compared to it. It is good to know the price which I pay for a beautiful orgasm, and that I have the choice if I want to pay it or not. Usually I do not feel like being totally worn out for two or three days due to having had an orgasm. So many big and small things have happened that I have for sure forgotten some of them.

Most importantly, my partner and I have come closer than ever before. Emotional moments have become more or more rare. We love to spend very, very much time with each other and have a hard time not being in each other's presence. That has been different in the past. We had moved into a bigger flat just because we could not stand it without each having a room on our own. And now we reorganized the flat and the single rooms have become a shared bedroom and office. This way we can always be in each other's presence and feel how the love is flowing forth and back.

My encounters with people are different. My heart is open. In the past I took a long time to find trust in someone. This now happens much more swiftly. My contact making is less language-oriented. I do not like talking as I used to. I prefer to be simply here, feeling inside of me and perceiving what is happening, instead of engaging in discussions. A lot of talking is strenuous for me and takes me away from myself. Whenever I had met a woman I did not yet know, an inner movie was going on: "We could have sex with each other. Do I want her? Does she want sex with me? But I have a girl friend. Bummer!" Now when I meet a woman I feel that my heart is open, that everything is OK, that I can talk with her and feel good. I have no need for sex as my imagination used to suggest it. I encounter the person in a way that has not been possible for me before. I really see her, instead of avoiding her in a way. Of course this does not always happen, but more and more often.

In the morning we both do exercises together. This gives me pleasure. And I am amazed how much this helps me to stay grounded in some critical moments. My need for a career, money, fame, appreciation, exciting journeys, meeting many friends has faded. I prefer to be with my beloved. And I am very content with that. If I could change my life from one day to the other, I would love to have a profession that allows me to stay at home every day, and not to travel around all the time. Recently we have been apart for ten days. And I easily loose the connection to my heart when I am alone. In the past I always wanted to be at home in order to come close to myself.

In the last month I woke up twice because I had an orgasm. I did not ejaculate. Ever since my puberty, I did not experience that. For one of these incidents I still recall that I had had a dream with wild sex fantasies. You had shared that it easily happens that you slip back into the conventional pattern. And we have short moments with a hot kiss, but the desire for hot sex is just there for a second and vanishes before we have the time to put it into practice.

I realized that my lust for sex has mutated into lust for life. Sometimes so much joy is bubbling up in both of us that we feel like exploding. My woman's menstruation is now normal, as it had not been regular for a very long time. And also she has a normal ovulation again. Best she will share this herself. We are very happy to have met you and very curious to see how everything will evolve. I can hardly believe that my life has changed so much in such a short span of time and in such a soft and harmonic manner. Thanks a lot.

Here come a few additions, in case you are interested in my experience. I find it unbelievable how much one can observe in respect to conventional sex.

Symptoms after the orgasm:

If I do not fall asleep right after the orgasm, and go for a walk, I have the following sensations:

- An intense idleness is spreading inside of me.
- Contact with people becomes difficult for me. I do not feel like seeing people.
- The front of my torso is extremely tense for the next two days.
- My lower back is contracted.
- My neck is tense.
- My body is generally tense. There is no space in me, no mobility.
- I am irritable.
- I behave like a child that did not have enough sleep, even if I slept a lot.
- Even little things are often too much. If I have to do something, it often feels like an insurmountable obstacle.
- My thoughts are racing.
- I doubt in my profession, my relationship, my living space, and my life. Nothing seems good as it is.
- I lack serenity. I feel no joy. I am afraid that everything will become too much.
- My eyes are blurred and my head feels foggy.
- I do not want to look at my beloved any more, and I am hardly able to look at her. And if I do it anyway, I do not

see her clearly.
- I feel restless.
- In brief, nothing is fun.
- I need about 2-3 days till I have recovered (at least), and I start watching movies endlessly and avoid contact.

Love, Kevin

Dear Kevin,
Thank you so much for the very interesting and thorough report of your experiences and insights. Discovering all this will certainly bring about a change in your life. And your report is particularly touching and convincing because of your young age – mid twenties. Perhaps your capacity to perceive this subtle level is because of your relative youth - compared to older people who have become more 'conditioned' and 'hardened' in their bodies and hearts. You have a heightened sensitivity and awareness that gives you insights through the ability to 'read' your own body and its reactions so well. Your words cause goose bumps on my skin and bring tears to my eyes. Best wishes to you both and may your life be filled with the joy of love.
Love, Diana

6. Experiencing that my fear is healed by love

Dear Diana,
With the tantric style of sex, I often realized how my love had the effect of me going beyond my personal self. The union of vagina and penis is firm as a rock, which keeps reminding me of my love.

As waves of emotion or fear threatened to overwhelm me, that genital connection helped me to stay aware of my love. With the help of love, I would then share my fear as opposed to being trapped in it and projecting it onto my wife. And, as we all know, the projection of fear is the most wonderful fertilizer for fights and separations.

Over all tantra has helped me a lot to deal with my patterns and fears. I can stay centered much better in myself when an old pattern comes up. I can name the patterns, and once they are out in the open on the table or in the bed, I can more easily deal with them constructively. Thank you for the tools!

Love, David

7. I get closed because I think my partner doesn't love me

Dear Diana,

I wanted to tell you about my being emotional! My problem in relationship is when I get closed because I think my partner doesn't love me really. **When I miss his attention then I start to play/act that I do not really need his attention, that I am very good on my own. And I start rejecting him because I want to punish him for not being nice enough to me.** Of course, that hurts him sometimes, but sometimes he is alert and he just stays with himself. That makes me see how childish I am, and sometimes it is not difficult to come out from this role.

The bigger problem is my insecurity in myself, judging the way I look, feeling that I'm not worthy. When I fall into this state, it is very difficult to come out of it. The roots of this thinking is in my childhood, because I was witnessing my parents' fights many, many times, and those fights were always about my father and other women. My mother was a very insecure person; her father left her and her mother, and she was afraid that my father would leave her too.

On the other side, my father really did have other women, and my mother was never sure about that, but she always attacked him with her suspicions. When I was about thirteen, my father was telling me stories about his love affairs with other women. So, inside me is a big mess. Sometimes when my partner and I are with some pretty woman, I just have an idea that he wants to be with her, and I become so jealous and scared and angry and sad that I just want to be alone; I do not want to have any contact with him.

I do the Osho dynamic meditation when that happens, and we talk about the situation afterwards and it helps. I have worked on this problem for years, and it is much, much better today (which means it doesn't happen very often), but it is still inside me. **Our doing tantric sex is sometimes also impossible when I feel like that, so I wanted to ask you – if I feel that way – sad, not worthy, I want to be alone, I think that all men are rubbish etc. – should we go into sexual contact or not?** We usually talk about my problems, but we do not bring our bodies together when this happens. My partner would like that, but I do not want to. What would you say about such a situation?

Love, Letitzia

Dear Letitzia,

Sorry to hear from you that you are having difficulties trusting the love of your man; that the old female conditioning of doubt and fear of losing love rises to the surface. It is sure to be part of your healing and cleansing. Certainly your mother's painful experiences that were witnessed by you as a child have had a strong impact on you, and so are coming up again and again. Jealousy and insecurity is a tough one, and I am speaking from experience; but it is something we have to overcome sooner or later. It is much easier to choose the path of emotion, than to stay centered in what is, present to what is. In fact we have to develop our inner male qualities in this direction.

In answer to your question, I would say that there is no rule to be made about whether it is good or not good to make love when you are feeling a bit disconnected. If it works and brings you closer, then it works, if it doesn't then it doesn't. It really depends how deeply you feel immersed in or identified with your emotions. Sometimes the 'wall' is there, yet slight, and coming into physical loving contact has the power to easily melt the feeling of separation or negativity.

So in that sense I feel bringing the bodies together, opening up to make love, is always worth it. And even when you are perhaps stuck a bit deeper in the emotions, having sexual contact can heal the disconnection. It really depends on the situation in hand, and I encourage you to experiment with it.

The touching thing is that your partner is ready to make love, even when you are a bit out of sorts, a sign that he loves you as you are. **There is really only one situation where I would say *not* to have sex, which is when a couple is in a highly emotional state and having an argument/or just finished one. Often the tension that remains in the body will move toward excitement and sex can easily become unconscious, hard and unloving.** So there is no real meeting and the seed of discontent is planted again and given more food. This is clearly not your situation, but since you ask about the issue of sex when a person is emotional, I thought I would add that for your interest. Wishing you love each day.

Love, Diana

8. I am desperate and I question my whole being as a man

Dear Diana,

I have wanted to write you for a long time about my joy and my experience as a man in the 'new' way of making love. Or, as we call it in the meantime, to 'be in love'. As it turns out, however, now I am writing to you in serious need, which I find a pity!

Since I participated in your Making Love Retreat a lot has changed regarding the way I make love, the way I look at making love, and in general the way I look at the sexual contact between men and women – it seems to me that it has changed not only for good (especially these last days). The worst thing I experience right now is that I do not feel anything anymore. I am not interested, I don't feel desire to be in love with my woman, at least not in sexual union. I do not even get visual stimulation any more when I gaze after young girls now and then. Yes, I don't even seem to be interested in stimulating myself. This makes me sad – actually, it frustrates me a lot.

It started slowly. After the seminar I was often excited before our making love appointments. I felt excited by that way of trying something new. I felt happiness because my partner likes this new way of making love so much. After a few weeks, we often noticed resistance before we headed towards the bedroom. One of us had a headache and the other was stressed from work, tired, or now the European Football Championship!

As soon as we had crossed that barrier, however, we both relaxed so deeply that I regularly fell asleep shortly after entering her and when I woke up I felt completely clear and fresh. During these first meetings I always had an erection before entering her, and when inside I felt delight and joy.

Then a time came when I did not have an erection anymore before making love. And as my penis is very small when it is not erect it became difficult to put it inside my woman (in the way you describe for soft penetration), sometimes even impossible. These situations frustrated me a lot. I did as you suggest when I became emotional. I told her I was emotional, I left the room, then shouted into several pillows, drank water and came back. Again I had no erection. (Ah, somehow it is difficult to write all that down.) I watched all this and thought to myself and talked to my partner that it was simply like this right now, not to worry, go on, it will change.

Then there were times when initially I had an erection but after entering I became so small again that my penis was not inside the vagina any more. And again the emotions came and also more and more frustration. My partner told me that it is not so important to her that I have an erection, she said that she even feels my penis more when he is not so hard and stiff. My fear of not having an erection, however, increased. The pressure even increased in a way that again, as I described earlier, there was no erection at all any more. And the frustration grew stronger.

Before the Making Love Retreat I thought that an erection was absolutely important for having sex. And that also the rhythmical movement was very important to sustain the erection. Because these goals were dropped, often when we were lying inside each other, I told my partner that I did not know what to do anymore, that it seemed almost boring to me. And I also fell asleep often. I was also careful not to move too much as I did not want to have an orgasm myself. And if we still ended up having one I somehow felt ashamed afterwards.

This is the situation I am in right now. I don't want to and I am afraid of making love again. My woman is sad because she benefits so much from making love in a new way and fears that it is over now. Right now I am really desperate and I completely question my whole being – in all life situations. And at the same time I know how important it would be right now to just lie down with my partner, have a massage, or listen to one of her fairy tales that she reads to me on those days of the month. **The issue with my very small penis is my primordial fear. And then, not even being able to make love causes a feeling of deepest shame. Shame and fear of woman. I feel the incredible pressure and the strong expectations that I burden myself with. Not only in love, in all of my life.** In theory I would know the answers that I would tell people in my situation, but right now I feel very alone with it and sad. Can you respond to my situation? Thank you.

Love, Christian

Dear Christian,

I am sorry to hear about your difficulties and challenges. During the retreat we do give you a completely different way of looking at sex and love, so it is a normal and a positive sign, that you have some kind of response or change of view in your life/sex. **That is the whole idea behind tantra – to learn how to transform sex into its higher vibration of love using the awareness. When you begin to have**

sex in a more conscious way a process of purification is set in motion. Any hidden or buried issues and emotions/feelings will surface as part of this cleansing and healing. For instance, the fears regarding erection, feeling ashamed of your penis, the sense that you do not know anything anymore, or becoming aware of the pressure you put yourself under in all parts of your life. All these aspects are very deeply rooted anxieties (in most men) that in the big picture have a draining effect on your life energy, which is also your sex energy. When these tensions begin to move (mostly in the form of emotions) you will of course begin to feel a bit negative and distant.

So it is good for you to realize that some of the things that you perceive as negative are actually to be viewed as positive! Even the fact that you do not look at young girls in the same sexual way actually reflects something going right with you and not something going wrong with you. When you do not look outward with sexually hungry eyes on young girls, this is indeed a relaxation for your life. Sex is ultimately an inner experience, dependent on a cellular vitality and not really to do with external visual stimulation and/or fantasy as we are led to believe/conditioned.

You will need to keep moving the waves of negative emotion out of your body by being physically active, in the way that you are already doing. **Attempt to transform the emotions into feelings, and allow yourself to feel what you feel, let tears flow if you can. Encountering and releasing any feelings of confusion, insecurity, or shame can be painful, however ultimately it will be healing and empowering.** Once you have allowed the tension to flow out of the body your outlook will immediately feel more bright and positive. Also you can begin to really involve yourself in your body and learn to be more present in it – whatever it is you happen to be doing. Maintain your body awareness during the course each day, how you sit, how you stand, how you eat, how you hug etc. Each day offers so many opportunities to 'feel into' the body. Anchoring yourself in your body and giving it a moment-by-moment value, will increase your presence and reduce the recurring negative thoughts. Do some exercise on a daily basis and you will feel an aliveness growing inside you that is wonderful and juicy and divinely sexual. Every time you make love, do some kind of movement/dance/exercise beforehand so that you become alive to yourself before you connect with your partner. Regular conscious body movement will also prevent a build-up of negativity and emotions. And at any time when you notice yourself a bit disconnected and negative, then move your body to get rid of this layer of tension. You are a young and beautiful man, and becoming more conscious in the body at this young age will be a great gift for your life.

Regarding not wanting to make love, this can be due to the layer of emotion that causes a sense of disconnection/negativity, but it can also be due to a bit of laziness on your part. Very often the resistance to sex is an unwillingness to be present per se, not actually a resistance to sex. To be present is an art and a challenge and the pleasures of it have to be discovered.

When you get together to make love be sure not to have rules, do not be black and white in your approach with fixed ideas of right or wrong. This is emphasized again and again during the retreat. For instance you say that you feel ashamed after having an orgasm – there is no need for this, nothing is wrong in it. It's just the *habit* of *always* wanting orgasm that is good to question. **The basic guideline we give you is that you make love with awareness, and that is all! Remember what was explained during the week – it is not *what* you do but *how* you do it. Anything and everything is fine provided it is conscious.** Stay alive to yourself but challenge your sexual habits at the same time. Awareness itself brings about powerful transformation.

Even when you do not feel like making love, make an inner commitment to having more love in your life, make dates with your woman, put your self into the situation, make a play of it, whatever happens is OK, cuddling, kissing or whatever. Just enjoy the simple being together without great expectations. It is possible to learn so much when two people are exploring within the same sexual frame. A great deal of healing and inner balancing becomes possible. And that transformation lasts for life; it is not only limited to this relationship. Your awareness and your body is with you wherever you go, and that means in the future you will be able to create loving situations with women.

Best wishes to you both.

Love, Diana

Dear Diana,

A quick note to say that your message made me feel much more relaxed and positive about my situation, thank you for that. And yes, you are right, I have definitely been struggling with my emotions! Incredible how they make me feel negative about life. I realized this several days before your message arrived, and started to work with my emotions in a constructive way so I am feeling much better and enjoying making love again!

Love, Christian

9. Sex is difficult for me because of high expectations and baby wish

Dear Diana,

My husband Axel and I participated in our first tantra seminar with you in May 2004 and it was a very beautiful experience for us. From then on, we have been experimenting quite a bit. Sometimes it was difficult for me. Sometimes it was completely relaxing and beautiful to get myself into love and tantra. In any case I have learned a lot since then. About two years ago we first wrote to you to tell you about our experience. And during last year while on vacation I read your new book *Tantric Orgasm for Women* and it opened up many things for me and confirmed that tantra is my way. I have wanted to write you to share my enthusiasm with you for some time now but somehow time passed and now I have a problem and need your help.

During the last month I have started to have difficulties with sexuality again. There are three things that play a role and they are intertwined. First, I frequently feel a wound in the area of my perineum and the pain inhibits my sensitivity and my relaxation because we have to interrupt the lovemaking. I feel guilty and responsible for it. Second, I have been in a conflict with myself and I still am. I did not know anymore what I really wanted exactly. During the last month I was more eager for conventional sex and for satisfaction or orgasm with clitoral stimulation and I was ashamed about it and I tried to suppress that energy or I only allowed it to happen once. I also realized that when I concentrate on my clitoris I don't feel the energy in my vagina anymore. Third and most important, for two years now we have wanted to conceive a child. Sometimes in times of stress and examinations I lost that wish. In the beginning we tried to plan and control but it did not work because I am very sensitive to pressure and I was no longer able to relax in love. I grew more and more convinced that the child would come when it wanted and that we could not control the conception. Axel did not agree and so we compromised to only partly control the situation. But that does not work either and neither do we make love regularly. In the last months, I have had the feeling Axel was only making love to me because of the wish for a child and somehow I felt exploited. Three weeks ago we had an important conversation about this issue after which we lay down together but I could not continue. In the conversation he had mentioned that he felt in a hurry because of our age (he will turn 39 and I will turn 36 soon). This made me very upset because I still think that we should not plan like this.

For me it is hard to find a balance between the wish for a child and sexuality, and in the end they belong together. Could you give me some advice on how to approach the whole thing more easily? What I suggested to Axel was that we first should try to make love without expectations so that penis and vagina could meet in a relaxed way again. What do you think?

I hope that the two of you are fine and I am looking forward to your reply.

Love, Hannah

Dear Hannah,

Thank you for writing, many things to say, I will try to keep it short and compact. Firstly, about the painful place that you are aware of on the perineum. This usually represents some kind of tension/wound/memory and can often be soothed and healed by placing the penis head directly on the pain spot. And then it is important that the man withdraw the penis a fraction so as to give a little space, being sure not to compact/compress the vaginal tissues. Remain present in this position and just be with the pain, allowing old feelings to surface and letting them move through you. Perhaps to refresh yourselves you can read again the chapters in the book/s about the deep penetration and relaxing and healing of painful places in the vagina.

Secondly, what I hear through your words is that quite possibly there are many feelings inside you that are not being expressed. There are many reasons why you may have these feelings, the child pressure, perhaps feeling a lack of love and intimacy, plus the disturbing pain in the perineum. Together these unexpressed feelings have possibly made you a bit 'low-grade' emotional. So it is good to check yourself on this level. I would suggest that the best way to move with these unexpressed feelings is to acknowledge that they are there, and then create a space to release them, take some time alone, allow yourself to weep, or be angry or whatever.

Thirdly, it has been my **observation, confirmed by many women, that when there is a gathering of unexpressed feelings, which means we are a bit 'emotional', we more easily become interested in the clitoris and the conventional way of sex.** This urge is usually an unconscious way to discharge the inner tensions instead of recognizing and dealing with the emotions directly. Perhaps this explains why recently you find yourself a bit more 'interested' in the clitoris. And anyway there is nothing wrong in being interested in the clitoris. We usually suggest to women who are 'interested' in the clitoris, that it is included more toward the end of lovemaking, rather than at the start. And the reason for this is precisely because of your observation – that you lose the connection to the vagina – after all, it is the receptacle for the penis and therefore very important to remain 'connected' to it.

So all your themes do hang together and perhaps the most direct way is to accept things the way they are, and do something physical (as mentioned already), or go to a therapist who works with the body, with breath for example, someone to help and support you.

Fourthly, I would suggest that perhaps you deal with the child wish by taking your daily temperature and begin to see when you are most fertile, and most likely to conceive. You will find books that explain this method. There are usually just a few days where fertilization can happen. On these days consciously go into sex with the idea of conceiving, getting pregnant, which means ejaculation.

Barry Long says that for conception the quicker the sex act the better. He says basically man should go in there and get the job done! Surprising isn't it? Anyway I trust him but you may want to read him yourself on this. He also says that woman should not try to have an orgasm herself, just to relax and receive. All this has an impact on the incoming soul, it is said. You can make a nice ritual, beautiful space, candles, flowers, music, a loving coming together and greeting etc., and then make the sex act quite simple. Afterward you can still lie together, united in the genitals, just being present together.

If you are able to isolate the days for 'getting pregnant', and focus on ejaculation specifically, then the other days of the month can be devoted to relaxed lovemaking with no fixed idea of orgasm or ejaculation in mind, and continue experimenting and creating love together.

I hope that your love wishes and your baby wishes can both be fulfilled in an effortless and joyful way.

Love, Diana

Dear Diana,

It's been a while since you answered me. I was very happy about your mail and I want to thank you for your support. It helped me and us a lot.

I saw a therapist that I know very well. During the session I realized that I had had a very high ideal with this issue and how the lovemaking should be when one wants to conceive a child. I thought it had to be very romantic and everything had to be perfect. All these expectations somehow instead created a distance to my wish for a child. When I read your mail I was fairly surprised that it can be so simple, without ceremony…

When you mentioned the temperature technique, I recalled that I once bought a little booklet about the temperature method. We both read it again. I felt open for it and was ready to give it a try. So we ordered the device and I am testing it now.

In the last two months we again 'paused' in our sexuality because I was very emotional. Axel and I will marry in April and I was panicking; fears and doubts came up. Now I know again what I want and we can start anew. It is such an exciting time! We are thinking about coming to the retreat again next year to get fresh impulses!

Many greetings.

Love, Hannah

Dear Hannah,

I am happy to hear that you are feeling more positive, allowing the dreams to come down to ground and see things in a more realistic light. It easily happens that we have high expectations (goals), and these do definitely stand in the way and 'block' what is! Yes, it will be valuable to come to the group a second (or third!) time, on each occasion you will experience it very differently. You will be more relaxed because you have done it before, but at the same time, because of your experience in between, you will hear and perceive everything on a deeper level. Best wishes to you and Axel for your marriage. Spring greetings to you both.

Love, Diana

10. Experiencing deep sadness and lethargy

Dear Diana,

First of all I want to thank you for your love, knowledge, calmness, and your wonderful way of conveying and living such special issues as sexuality and love. The week with you fulfilled a long-time wish for me. When I met my lover three and a half years ago I found your book by chance exactly during the same first days and I thought it was the cure for all my apparent "problems". Problems as you describe them: lack of passion, inner distance etc. In the first six months we had rather hot sex of course, but then we experimented with the help of the book and I was able to get an idea of what you are talking about. We moved in together and daily routine entered life and bedroom and just like many times before I felt as if behind a wall, longing for caring tenderness, closeness and connection. My partner wanted the hot sex that we had in the beginning...

To cut the long story short: finally we came to your retreat and we were both astonished how easy it actually was to feel something completely different. Closeness, tenderness... and having sexual feelings at the same time... for sure the week was not always easy for us, but we came closer again and I feel that many things do not scare me that much any more. Now we are back home and also here we try to practice and to find spaces in the daily routine. We manage fairly well.

There is one thing I cannot explain though: Since we returned I feel worse and worse. **I feel extremely sad inside but I cannot cry and I do not know why I feel this way. I feel heavy as if I had been ill for a long time. I do not want to do anything. Everything feels like a burden. Taking a walk, riding the bike - puh - pure effort. My lower back hurts from bending my legs so much and the "old" tensions in the shoulder girdle are worse than before. I have headaches as if I was sitting at the desk all the time.** It feels as if everything was horrible, but right now things are going great (even the other issues like money, school, living etc. are currently not horrible for a change!) Do you know this? It tortures me to see all the good, all the beauty and not being able to feel it at all!

I keep on telling myself that things are great - and? Nothing. Just a deep sadness, as if I was feeling lovesick. As if something was missing. And I do not even have an idea what it could be!? It feels strange. So today I decided to write you and I would be very happy to receive an answer!

Love, Helena

Dear Helena,

Firstly let me thank you for your presence in the retreat – your radiance and love was a like a silent ocean of support – to see and feel your beauty, inner and outer.

As to your sharing and query about your experience of deep sadness and complete lethargy since the retreat – this is very real and a sign of deep purification happening on a cellular level. **Bringing consciousness into the sexual channel displaces old stuff, personal and collective, which accumulates unconsciously in the body. Many of us carry the sadness for the whole of humanity, and it may be necessary on your journey to allow the sadness and the tears. You may have to cry for hours and hours, even days, following the wisdom of the body.** As you say, it is not all that easy, but for sure you can create the space intentionally, and put aside 2-3 hours so that you can go deeply into the feelings. Play music that touches your heart and soul, relax into your body, and allow yourself to feel, give way and surrender to any and all the sadness, encouraging tears to flow and cleanse your system. The tiredness you are experiencing can be due to the effort of holding these feelings down, or repressing them.

Another source of the bone-tired feeling is because when relaxation enters the sex center, which is at the basement of the system, all the old exhaustion comes to the surface. Most of us have been involved in doing much too much all these years, with inadequate rest and relaxation. Beautiful if you can give yourself space and accept the situation, welcome the discomfort knowing that the old has to move so as to make way for the new. If while you are making love any sadness arises, then give way to it, make a passage for it, and you can remain together in the sexual connection that is initiating the cleansing and the healing. Love, Diana

Dear Diana,

I am deeply touched by both of you and very grateful for everything you have said, done and shared - even without words. Now I want to quickly tell you how life has continued for me. I am not that lethargic and the sadness is not that present anymore but I was not able to "really" cry recently. My heart is still in turmoil and deep inside the sadness is still there!

Well, of course in the meantime everything has changed again. My "last" comfort is always that I know now that nothing stays/remains as it is - above all not feelings. Slowly, slowly the work of the daily routine catches up with us and it gets harder to find space for longer practicing times. But for now we continue to work on what was started in the retreat and I hope that it will turn into a stable foundation.

Last Wednesday my partner and I had a severe discussion - in bed - and afterward I was able to cry a little but somehow the sadness is still blocked. It will come when the time is right: I am absolutely open for it! Indeed, last Wednesday was very sobering for me. It was already last Sunday that my partner said he wished for a more active sexuality and on Wednesday he really challenged it. We had a date for making love and it was clear what he wanted. Today he wanted passion, kissing, sex. I was in shock almost immediately. This had been our problem before Easter as well - he wanted sex more often and more heavily and I did not. And now I could not go with it. We started a discussion (yes, I know, we should have separated...) that ended in my partner saying his needs were not fulfilled but only mine and that this was not OK for him. After all, women were to prepare the emotional soil and to invite and help men.

How much I wished you were there. It was so hard for me to stay loving with him and myself. Unfortunately the last times (before Wednesday) were not especially intense or exciting. We plugged in and moved a little - but somehow there was no energy. It is really difficult to create or keep this energy in normal life.

I realized that I was overwhelmed by his comment on the emotional soil. I do not really know what I am supposed to do about it. There is a huge difference for me in feeling, just being there, breathing, and a manipulative, fascinating way of goal oriented physical lust where you are still caught in your own space as if you are masturbating on the other. For me this is not "love". **But how can I find the middle between both poles? I do not want my partner to feel a lack. I understand him well. He loves his power and energy - and he loves it most in sex with intense movement. I simply feel unable to make the connection. As soon as he moves more and gets excited every-thing inside of me closes as if I had to protect myself.** We did not practice the last two days. Sunday we will have our next date and I am curious what will happen then.

Ah, dear Diana, it would be so nice to have women circles where we could talk about these things. We are all in different situations and it could support me to hear about the experience of others. But I do not want to complain. I am happy and grateful that I have at least one woman - you - one that I can tell all this to...!

I would be very happy to receive an answer!

Love Helena

Dear Helena,

I am sorry to hear that you are experiencing a phase of feeling challenged because of a difference of 'intention' as far as making love goes. This can easily happen even if we are inspired by a uplifting tantric vision - because actually putting it into practice for real comes with its challenges, and you are facing one at present. Important is how you deal with it. If you get emotional or generally feel a bit prickly or 'over sensitive' or reactive (as symptoms of emotion) then it is a great support to do something with the body on a daily basis, and also suggest your partner does the same. Moving the body on a regular basis serves to balance you by burning up the subtle tensions of accumulating emotion. You will always notice that after a series of exercises or body movement your whole psyche is more positive, and your sense of your body heightened.

Very often, it is in fact the pressures, stresses and tensions of the work and survival that cause us to be somewhat 'emotional'. This underlying tension that many of us carry can be the reason why people become drawn/impelled toward climax, because through the climax inner tensions are discharged. On a superficial level there appears to be a type of 'relaxation' after a climax, but on a deeper level some tension remains in the system because tension itself was involved in the build-up to the climax. So the end result is tension, and not true relaxation

Moving your bodies regularly will deal with any the accumulated tensions, giving them another outlet, and then restlessness will not enter the lovemaking so easily. Added to this, it is quite usual that the normal conditioning hangs around for a while, raises itself, shows itself; it is part of the process of deconditioning ourselves, and especially men due to their heavy conditioning to do/perform in sex. So there has to be some bridging, some allowing for experimentation, some focusing on yourself and seeing what you can do to transform the situation through your awareness, relaxation and presence rather than focus on how he is not doing it right. This shift will make all the difference to your experience.

At the same time it is helpful to realize that when we are a little bit upset as you may be at the moment (a bit in an emotional state, finding 'fault' with the other, focused on the outside), this will make you a bit tense and influence your receptivity, because your are not resting with your awareness fully rooted inside of your body/being. Remember receptivity is a force and it can transform what enters the field. Your presence on a cellular level can slow your man down, bring him into the present, so first look to see what you can do from your end whenever possible. When man is made to feel wrong with every move he makes then for sure he gets more identified with his usual way. We teach tools and not rules. For exploration to have depth there needs to be some level of co-operation, and I am sure if you are patient, compassionate, loving, and maintain a sense of humor, then things will change by themselves.

Love, Diana

11. Feeling more often frustration and boredom

Dear Diana,

It has been two months since the wonderful and very valuable seminar in Germany and we want to share our first experiences in every day life.

In the meantime for both of us the initial enthusiasm for the new style of making love has turned into frustration and boredom more often. It is true that we made progress together and that the new style of making love has brought us closer together which is good for our relationship. More closeness, love, trust, exchange and commitment has grown between us. In general our relationship has improved and become "wider". Joachim does not have pain in his testicles anymore when he does not ejaculate. He feels more relaxed in his pelvis area and his erection feels "softer yet fuller". Anna feels more in her vagina. The connection to the breasts improves slowly, but often she does not really feel connected to her positive pole, not really at home in her breasts. A feeling of energy and overflow is not there yet.

You might want to know that we mostly meet on weekends to make love once or twice. However, we have been repeatedly frustrated and bored.

Why are we not happy? What makes us wondering?

- We both had a genital fungal infection
- An occasional burning sensation in the vagina despite a lot of oil
- Mostly a tight and tense vagina
- Till now when making love we have avoided lust, excitement, and go for what we think ecstasy is (to stay in the cool zone)
- Sometimes we do not take the two or three hours when making love
- Often there is a goal orientation in our ideas and expectations – probably the reason for frustration and boredom because "nothing really happens"
- When Joachim's erection weakens (without we have not yet managed a penetration) we both feel nothing or only very little and this often causes boredom. We change position and start with a new erection but after that very quickly we are bored again and sometimes disappointed and frustrated.
- When Joachim loses his erection he feels impotent and not as a man.
- We wished for a more fulfilled sexuality but we have not yet really found it.

We would be very happy to receive feedback. With your experience and knowledge, what do you think about our situation?

I hope you are fine, enjoying the wonderful summer... wherever you are.

Lots of love

Anna & Joachim

Dear Anna & Joachim,

To my ears, it sounds like everything is going perfectly well at your end. It just depends on how you view the situation. The best you can tell us is that the ambience of love and harmony is alive and well, even though there may be some frustration arising in the lovemaking. But this is secondary really. Most important is that you are experiencing a deepening in love through the awareness you have been bringing into your being together. When we enter the tantric realm, we are transforming ourselves, not only improving our sex lives.

It is quite possible that you experienced fungus infections as part of a clearing and cleansing. If infections continue to occur it is advisable to go to a doctor, and/or look at your diet, and ways to reduce the acidity of the body, drink lots of water etc. Also monitor the emotional part of yourselves. Are you keeping yourselves free in the solar plexus? Are you expressing your feelings and not getting emotional?

For a man to experience his 'loss of manliness' through loss of erection is for sure difficult, but when he can just relax into the situation, accept what is happening, and allow the erection to go down (rather than try to stimulate himself into erection again), ultimately it is an integrating and profoundly healing experience. There may be feelings of helplessness or weakness – just feel what is present without judging it or trying to change it. If tears wish to flow, don't hold them back. If the body starts shivering or shaking, co-operate with it. Allowing unexpressed feelings that may have been hidden for a lifetime is an empowerment, and through this process slowly man becomes more of man – with a true male authority, a man who knows and accepts and trusts himself in his depth.

As to your frustration and boredom, this is entirely your choice, you are creating the situation and therefore you can change it. It is up to you each as individuals to remain alive to your bodies. You can do some exercises or dance movement to awaken your body energies before connecting.

Perhaps you have made too much of a concept of 'how' lovemaking should be, instead of making love, and remaining

as conscious and present as possible each time! And it requires time and practice to step down from the ingrained patterns and habits.

So, yes, I would definitely say that you are *very* impatient, busy looking for results and not appreciating the gifts on the journey of transformation (for example – that you generally feel more loving with each other), you do not allow any unfolding...

There is a tendency for the mind to habitually look toward the negative, and to disregard/take for granted the positive. When the positive is not consciously given enough value then that leads to an over-emphasis on the difficult aspects. Perhaps you have this mindset a little, which means you are not really appreciating how much has changed in the last weeks. Remember you are overturning a very old conditioning and time in years is needed, as well as a lot of real clock time spent in making love!

And think in terms of an ongoing adventure rather than looking for immediate results, with a goal to be reached. There is no goal at all; in fact the way is the goal. And to be 'present' cannot be a goal, because your body is already in the here and now, it is more a matter of you realizing it and appreciating it. **Really in the ten weeks or so since we met each other, you have done extremely well, and honestly, ten weeks is a drop in the ocean of experience...**

I suggest that you read and read again, Osho or Barry Long or any of our books, so that you can stay inspired and also have some insights into your experiences. As your experiences deepen so will your understanding. Congratulations for your sincerity and efforts in love. I wish you a loving summer.

Love, Diana

Dear Diana,

Thank you so much for your feedback. Again it was very helpful and took away our frustration. We had completely forgotten that lovemaking should be fun as well. Anyway we are determined to continue on the tantric path. We will see were the journey wants to take us. Much love to you.

Anna & Joachim

12. I really have no clue how to deal with my 'blocks'

Dear Diana,

Thank you for your offer to keep contact! I write now because I feel a little 'helpless' in how to continue with what we experienced in The Making Love Retreat. I haven't seen my partner very much, since we do not live in the same city. We made one date, starting with a massage, but afterwards we both felt unhappy.

There was this heaviness between us. I think I again had the attitude to 'make things work', but I was making it, forcing it, not feeling it. I really have no clue how to deal with my 'blocks', the 'no' to penetration and how to be in a relationship. And how I can learn not to be too serious about it. I want to be 'a good girl'– but it doesn't work this way (luckily). So I am standing here with a big question mark. If you have any ideas about this I would appreciate it.

Love, Gisela

Dear Gisela,

I am not sure what to suggest to you at this moment because your situation is delicate owing to your history of sexual abuse that has made you particularly sensitive to the approach of a man. And this is very understandable. On the one hand, it is good to honor and respect the body, to listen to the 'no' rather than force a 'yes'. But at the same time sex is a healing force (when rightly employed) so there is also a value in challenging oneself, knocking on the door, without pressure and 'I must', but with curiosity and asking 'who am I'. I was very touched at the end of the group when you came up to me and said that you realized that you do not 'know' yourself. Because your insight is the truth, we do not truly 'know' ourselves as human beings.

And the basic reason is because we do not know our sexual selves and our sexual beings. When we discover the natural sexual intelligence that lies in the body, the complimentary polarities of the body and between bodies, we come to know ourselves better, feel more grounded, rooted, more present, more confident, more in love, and it becomes much more easy just to 'be'.

I suggest that you do not focus on whether you want penetration or not, the yes or the no of it. See what happens, and go with the flow, no pressure either way. What can be more interesting for you is to monitor/keep checking your level of emotionality, noticing if you feel connected/disconnected, can look in the eyes/or not – you remember the symptoms of emotions we talked about in the group. Sometimes there is even a state of low-grade emotionality, which is a bit like a low-grade infection, where a person can feel a little bit blue, little bit depressed, a bit disconnected basically all the time. Check this level of reality out. Whenever you find you are 'emotional' even if on a *very* subtle level, do something about it, move the body etc. Also when you are together with your partner keep checking what is happening behind the scenes.

Often a store of unexpressed feelings in the body can cause the resistance to wanting to open up. So it is not you that cannot open up, but the tension of the unexpressed feelings lying in between that you are feeling act as a barrier. These are creating the resistance and it is helpful to reach them and release them consciously. You can set aside some time, put on some heart opening music, and have a good weep, let the sadness flow through you. It may take a few hours. Or you may have to do create this space for yourself a few times. Whenever you feel unhappy, allow the tears. After the massage when you both felt unhappy, it also represented a moment to get into the old feelings, wash them away with tears, leaving you cleansed and more available to the moment.

I am suggesting only that you stay fresh with yourself, observe your emotional level, and work with your body consciously to disperse emotions. It sounds like hard work, but not really, because the pleasure and lightness of being which follows is worth it. I suggest you do some exercise routine every day because this can help tremendously to reduce the subtle gathering of emotions.

The fact that your partner lives a distance from you is a disadvantage because of the expectations and pressures that something has to happen in the short periods when you are together. But at the same time different cities gives you space apart from him, time all for you. Which is also a gift. It means that when you do see each other you are fresh, not in any routines or taking each other for granted. As I perceive your man he is a loving, patient, sincere being and I feel certain that he will walk by your side through the difficulties; doing so will certainly making him more grounded in his male authority, his love, his compassion, and his ability to be present with what is.

The situation you are in is delicate and the best you can do is let it be a dance, rather than a problem. At the end of the day only you can know what is right for you and when it is right for you. You have to use your intelligence. You will find listening to the Barry Long audio CDs on Making Love, and reading Osho, a great support and will give you ongoing encouragement, inspiration. Meditating on your breasts, melting into them and loving them, will help you to become more rooted in your body, and your femininity. I do hope that these few words can be of some support to you.

Love, Diana

Dear Diana,

I was very happy to get your answer, thank you! We have been on vacation in between, and that was not so easy in terms of emotions. Now back to daily life I watch myself avoiding the issue a little bit. Your suggestion about checking the level of emotion is helpful for me. Yes, there is this subtle state of feeling a little depressed. I am now experimenting with exercises and movement always to keep myself more in touch with my body-self.

Last weekend we had a good time, very playful, also making

love. My partner was so sweet and loving, it was great. I felt a bit 'dirty' afterwards which was strange, so I had to take a shower. I think it was some kind of cleansing of memories from the past. But it was still nice and deepened our connection. **Often I am not able to clearly see or feel the subtle emotional state, or what emotion is behind. I don't feel the sadness or whatever is there. It feels more 'diffused'.** I do not know how to deal with this. Anyway, the week with you was a challenging and a nourishing experience, and one that I would not want to have missed!

Love, Gisela

Dear Gisela,

Thank you for letting me know how you are getting along. To me your process sounds to be going in the right way, subtle shifts and changes, increasing the flow of love between you. When things change slowly the changes are for real; they reflect a shift in consciousness. You are on track if you stay with your body as much as possible, and continue to do body things. **It is really not very important to understand what emotions/and why emotions. If you have an insight, if understanding comes to you, then that is good. But if there is no insight, then that is also good.** If you notice that you feel disconnected, even on a subtle level, then get your body moving, and it is perfect that you are doing regular daily movement. This will help disperse the subtle build up of emotions.

For you (and all of us!) the body is the key, and helps you to shift your focus away from the mind and thought, to connecting with the simple here and now. We are pleased to hear that the week was of value to you. Best wishes to you both.

Love, Diana

13. These old emotions are somehow 'sitting' on my sexuality.

Dear Diana,

I am writing to share an interesting observation: A woman came for a massage and almost at the end of the massage she got in touch with a deep pain and sadness. I was just present with her and not asking too much; she was talking just a little bit about it. When the session was over I got in touch with my emotions of a deep sadness too. Somehow I knew that it had something to do with my old wounds but I didn't know. I remembered that you also said during the workshop that it's not always necessary to know the reasons, but that it is absolutely necessary to move the body. So I did and some of the pressure from my solar plexus dissolved. What I found out is this, that after releasing these emotions, I felt a soft flow of energy through my body, a light feeling of sexual energy in my body, mainly in the breasts and the lower part of the belly. It looks like these old emotions are somehow 'sitting' on my sexuality. I hope this is true and not only because at the moment I am in the state of ovulation. Yesterday my partner and I had a very good talk about all this and at first he was telling me about himself, how he feels at the moment with his sexuality and then afterwards we made love. I was not able to put my partner's penis in without an erection because my vagina was still very tight, but with an erection we were able to find a very nice soft approach again, without stimulation and orgasm, and afterwards we both felt very nourished. I definitely felt my vagina much more sensitive and open after releasing the emotions! What a miracle!

Love, Almira

Dear Almira,

Thank you so much for sharing your experiences. And it is so good that you did not feel the need to understand 'why' or 'what' comes to the surface, and let yourself get distracted by trying to analyze the situation, but just to support the wave to move through you. Your insight that followed is really profound in that it is absolutely true that our old pains are tensions that 'sit on' our sexuality, and ultimately make us less sensitive. So when the tensions move out of the system, all the cells are refreshed and revitalized, as evidenced by the soft flow of sexual energy you could feel in your body afterwards. I am sure that as you continue making love, allowing old feelings to arise, you will soon feel the vagina becoming more relaxed and sensitive.

Best wishes.

Love, Diana

14. Our journey with love and letting go of emotions

Dear Diana,

It has been almost a week since the week in Germany with you and the effects are *enormous*! I feel so great, calm and much more. Considering the "greater whole" of humanity I am writing to share my experience with (almost) these few words. On my healing path I have done sooooo many things in the last nine years, always hoping and looking for healing which I gradually found. However, since last week I feel that I haven taken *huge steps in the right direction*. I feel so peaceful and calm and relaxed. Not to mention what has opened up in me, and could open up between Hans and me.

Your work is wonderful and the mind does not have to ask if this is the truth because you are the message. Thanks a million!

Love, Sigrid (& Hans)

Dear Sigrid,

Thank you for your loving message. It is wonderful to hear that you are experiencing the enriching effects of the retreat, and all due to your own sincerity and receptivity. Having a new orientation in love is sure to open up the way for a simpler sweeter life, day by day. Best wishes to you both.

Love, Diana

Dear Diana,

Hans and I are still great. *We are full of gratitude* (and I almost have tears in my eyes writing this). We have a great life with and in the "cool zone". The changes are so peaceful. I feel completely relaxed. It is unbelievable. **At the same time I have been struggling with restlessness, anxiety, a very familiar nausea, and dizziness in the last week. Sometimes I literally get afraid of how much has changed in my world regarding sex. Is it maybe connected to the abuse?** I know this condition but have not had it for months. Now it happens almost every morning after I wake up, after dreaming. I do not take it too seriously and tell myself that it is maybe still my insecure inner child who cannot trust that much peace, closeness, and trust in Hans...? Sometimes I was overwhelmed by the fear if this new sexuality will really work after living it so differently sooo many years. I think I "just" need a little more time to digest everything and to be able to believe that this kind of sexuality is also nice for Hans, to trust that he "does not miss anything" (his words!).

Sigrid

Dear Sigrid,

It is heart-warming to hear that you experience peacefulness and relaxation through being more aware and cool in sex. To me these are indications that you are definitely on track. Part of the purification process is that unresolved issues, the memories, the doubts or negativity will come to the surface, so while it may be uncomfortable it helps if you understand why it needs to happen. Memories relating to your abuse will also be cleansed from the system so the more you can accept the situation, the easier it is going to be. If you can take some 'distance', and not get too identified with the situation, that will help you.

You now know that there is definitely another way and you need to trust this, together with your experience so far, and remembering that 'afterwards is your teacher'. It is really a great moment when your man tells you that he 'misses nothing'; it will make it easier to open new doors and help to step away from the conditioned sex. And to have a man that is willing is a tremendous relaxation for you, and a blessing.

Love, Diana

Dear Diana,

Some time has passed since we met the second time in a group. Now I want to tell you quickly about our highlight... It was in bed yesterday evening when a normal conversation lead to an argument. He discussed, I discussed. He got angry and I gave him the "time-out sign" (to which we had agreed upon) and after a few minutes he got up "nicely angry" and **said the famous seven words: "OK, I am emotional. I am coming back." This was *totally* liberating for me. *Finally, finally, finally* I did not feel like "being silenced". Ten minutes later he was back and five minutes later we embraced again.** We will even manage to make the issue of emotions easy.

Yes, and then when we made love I suddenly felt a *new sensation* inside of me. I do not care if it was ecstasy or not. It was just wonderful. It came by itself and stayed several minutes. My problem was "only" that it scared me. It was *wonderful* but it felt rather unpredictable. And it did not stop as fast as a usual orgasm either. It felt quite uncontrollable. Afterward I felt great but I was a bit nauseous until the morning, a bit overwhelmed, a little confused...

However, I think that this will pass and that some day it will no longer scare me.

Indeed, we are very grateful that our love can blossom more and more with your "love keys", that more and more barriers in our hearts disappear and that we can come really *close* to each other. And really many thanks to you again.

Have wonderful summer days.

Sigrid

Dear Sigrid,

It was a real pleasure to meet you and Hans again, to feel how your connection, love and awareness have deepened in the year between the two Making Love retreats. Also during the group to see and feel your commitment to love, and your courage to face old emotional patterns very directly. Important is that you allowed the process to unfold further at home in an intelligent way, compliments! The experience you describe is really groundbreaking and will give you a totally new feeling for your body. The nausea that you felt afterwards, also the confusion you felt, is part of the purification and integration. During the group, you both looked wonderful, beautiful, and radiant - a reflection of the beauty of your beings...

Love, Diana

Dear Diana,

You probably receive mostly positive mails from people, and I have been writing you from cloud nine so far as well. Now, however, it seems that Hans and I cannot find each other any more since I "realised my conditioning" during the follow-up days with you in December. Back then I said that I did not yet know where recognising this pattern would lead me, what to do with it. I was still a little bit confused. It is true that it has brought me closer to myself but not closer to Hans. I just do not want any arguments or discussions anymore. And maybe we are actually really too different. In fact, the last four years of our relationship were not so easy. But love made us stay together all the time. But now I am asking myself if I want this when it leads to these arguments again and again. I come to my borders. My body shows me clearly that it is not good for me when I cannot eat or sleep. I love so much what you teach and I know that this is my path.

It is so hard for me to stand harshness in a relationship if it is *close*. I can be harsh with myself but if I live in a close relationship with *love* I can hardly stand harshness. This closeness that Hans and I share and then again and again this harshness where my heart bleeds... And now, already since November/December 2008 I feel that my heart stays closed. It just does not want to open again in this relationship. The hurts have left their traces. I long for calmness and peace and I look for it by increasingly spending time alone. I do the Five Tibetan exercises every day and try to find out what is good for me. The more I am true to myself the more I distance myself from Hans. This is a pity. I am curious to see if the situation will change for a better and we find each other again or if we will separate. Somehow I wanted to write you for some days now to tell you what is going on with us, with me. Greetings to both of you and lots of love!

Sigrid

Dear Sigrid,

I am sad to hear that it has not been such an easy time for you. At the moment, it is good not to do anything about your situation, do not try to decide what to do. Just let it be, relax with it and do not think too much about if you must stay or go, and all the problems of the last four years. **Too much thinking/ thoughts/mind has the power to create subtle emotions, which make you feel in a fog or disconnected.** Try to stay with the simple joy of each movement or activity. Use your body as a bridge to the simple 'now' moment. When you find your mind circling around with negative thoughts, see if you can replace them with uplifting positive thoughts.

You can make it a daily practice; to take some moments to feel grateful for the blessings life is giving you, the life with Hans, the love with Hans, all the learning. Forget about the future, live today. And never forget that you and Hans have had difficulties because of your having his children living with you, which has made the years more of a challenge.

I can only encourage you to stay on track, taking small steps at a time.

Love, Diana

Dear Diana,

I just got up to send you an email and there was your reply! Thank you so much for it. We have to encourage ourselves again and again to stay on track. Again and again one of us doubts and this is not good at all! I do not want to think or talk about "leaving or staying" but it still happens. This is a pity. I feel so much love inside of me and that makes me happy. It makes me happy that I never lost love. Even though it sometimes hides behind a hard crust... I will not lose it anymore. It is there in my daily routine and it makes me grateful.

Love to you and thank you so much for your message, for your help. I am really very glad to know you. It is a beautiful and honest path towards where I *always* wanted to be, already as a child: calmness, peace, honesty between people and warmth and love. A warm embrace

Love, Sigrid

Chapter 4

Sexual Subjects

1. No feeling and a loss of energy

Dear Diana,

My husband has a question. When we try to make love with soft penetration and he has no orgasm he says he feels *nothing* during the penetration. And he wonders why not because I am tingling with energy feelings right through my body, and down my arms and legs. He does not have this. He feels himself without energy and power the whole day if we managed to make love in the morning. Then at night it happens that he cannot sleep because he has *too* much energy in his system. I feel myself safe and glorious, filled with energy and happy.

Why does he have the feeling that he gives all his energy to me?

Love, Angela

Dear Angela,

It is a very common situation that a man will, in the beginning, have some difficulty in sensing his genitals from a more internal perspective. Initially it's a step down from a hot active style to a cool relaxed style, from sensation to sensitivity, so some time and space for adjustment must be allowed for. There is bound to be a gap in experience. In fact you are entering a process where there will be constant changes, and it is good to be curious and just observe without making quick conclusions or getting over-identified with what happens. **Engaging more consciously in sex does and will have cleansing effects on the whole system; even if a person may feel nothing on the surface, on a more profound level there will be an effect that will ripple through. Relaxing in the sex center brings up many old buried tensions/issues for purification.**

So the fact your husband feels without power or energy can also be seen in a positive light. Nothing is going wrong. And layer by layer old tensions, memories, anxieties are cleansed from the body and psyche as an essential part of healing and transformation. When he later in the day experiences too much energy, and can't sleep, this is definitely not a problem either. He must enjoy being awake and find ways to use his energy creatively. He will sleep when his body really needs to. As far as I can tell, everything seems to be evolving in a balanced way. It is most helpful for him to allow any old unexpressed feelings that come to the surface. Honor and trust the body, and surrender to the flow. In these ways we become more pure, the psyche more clear, and the body more sensitive.

There is no question of your husband giving up his energy or his power to you. You do not take anything away from him.

In fact, he is experiencing a cleansing of some kind that is ultimately empowering. It is also quite normal that a woman is able 'to feel' more easily than man. Woman, as the more receptive, feminine pole, is much more likely to have a sense of what enters inside her. She is the surrounding, the ambience, and therefore more easily aware of what enters or moves through her space. And it helps man to hear from you what *you feel in your vagina*/body; your words will give him more confidence and trust in himself. There is some relaxation in realizing that even if he can't (yet) feel himself, at least you can feel him. There is going to be some type of energetic exchange due to the presence of the male pole inside woman's body. The penis will be a trigger for all kinds of energy flow, but the ultimate sensitivity and inner energy streaming is yours as an individual.

Man often feels less because the usual style of sex has a desensitizing effect on the penis. Through the stimulation it gets a bit tense and overcharged. And usually there will be a basic disconnection from the body tissues, especially the web of muscles that surround and form the genitals. In this area, called the pelvic floor, there is a general deadness, lack of vitality and awareness. On a physical level a man can do a great deal to remedy the situation through increasing his own body awareness. He can and should inwardly bring attention to his perineum and anus, and relax the area, as many times a day as he can manage, and whenever he remembers. And this little awareness exercise can be done in any situation, because it's not visible to others.

Receiving massage on the buttocks, thighs, calves, legs and feet is very supportive and helps a man to ground his energy. People can also do much good for themselves through self-massage – massaging their own legs and feet. Regular exercise is a great help. A man has to learn to focus his awareness on a subtle vibrant vitality that exists in the body. It means bringing the perception down to the cellular level and becoming his penis, rather than using his penis, and this is a journey that needs time and, above all, lots of practice and patience.

Love, Diana

2. Dealing with moments of nothingness

Dear Diana,
Your explanation (above 1.) makes it more clear what is happening for us. I notice the most difficult aspect for my husband is *when* he feels nothing. Because of this he avoids making love. How can he deal with his nothingness?

Love, Angela

Dear Angela,
There can be fear in relation to the experience of 'nothingness'; it can be like a small 'death'. At the same time, deep transformation is possible when a person (man or woman) simply relaxes and falls into an acceptance of not feeling anything. Just to be with that and to say yes to what is, instead of fighting and denying it, wanting things to be different. These kinds of tensions will actually stop a person from feeling. Acceptance enables tensions to flow away, brings deep relaxation and will increase the capacity to 'feel'. (It may help him to express in words how he feels when there is just 'nothing', and to allow any wave of old unexpressed feelings that follow.) There needs some willingness to be 'in the gap'. So in this sense it is best for a person to stop looking and expecting to feel something, but instead relax back into himself, and just 'be'. Resting with attention within the body in a more receptive mode, present to *what is* instead of putting the focus on *what is not*. Worse case scenario is that even if your partner feels nothing at least he is lying in his bed, and with you, and inside you – what a heavenly situation. It's the expectations that get in the way, and the pressure to get it right immediately.

Having said all the above, if you husband feels 'nothing' he can also move a bit, until he can feel 'something'. It's good to climb down slowly from the mountain, and not try to be resting in the valley immediately. In this sense woman needs to be a 'bridge' for a man, with a bit of give and take, even though she may prefer a more still style of making love right away. But stillness must not be made into a rule or a technique; it is only one option, and one that you grow into. Most significant is that man is conscious and present to woman when he is inside her. There are choices in life that mean we may need to become awkward beginners all over again, where a blend of intelligence, curiosity and courage is needed.

After making love it is a good idea to remain in bed for twenty minutes and enjoy simply resting. Lie on your backs, parallel but without any physical contact, keeping the head, neck and spine in one line. Legs extended, and place a pillow underneath the knees. Bring your attention into your own bodies and allow the cellular experience —whatever it is – to continue moving inside you. 'Being' like this will help to anchor you in the body, and give you the opportunity to tune into the subtle sensations of the inner world. And in moments when you are filled with awareness, in a state of relaxation and pure presence, boundaries dissolve, you become filled light – and this is pure bliss.

Love, Diana

3. Valuing my vagina over clitoral stimulation

Dear Diana,

I have a question for you that I think you will be able to answer. Your book was so resonant with my sexuality and I've *never* read anything that felt so 'right on' – and I've read a lot. Especially the way you speak of the breasts and vagina. So here is my question. Very personal, but I know this is your realm. I have found that *all* of my orgasms (and I am an ejaculator since I was 19 years old) are vaginal, and very deep. I feel like I don't even need my clitoris, so much so that when it comes to oral sex for me, it practically puts me to sleep. I find it soothing, and not stimulating. What are your thoughts on that, as my partners have always loved doing that, but it bothers them that it shuts down my fire?

Love, Beatrice

Dear Beatrice,

Your orientation on the vagina is just perfect. It's more a question of man (and woman) being re-educated. Your observation certainly accords with the way the female body is designed. **Woman's deepest orgasms emanate from the depth of the vagina, and not through the clitoris.** I understand full well your lack of interest in the clitoral stimulation of oral sex, and that it can also be a bit of a turn-off. This is something I realized shortly after I began to have sex as a teenager; so like you, I have since been oriented on my vagina and not my clitoris.

Clitoral stimulation engages the energy on a superficial level because it tends to takes the direction of excitement/orgasm etc. However, both men and women are conditioned to believe that the clitoris is the center of female sexuality and the source of satisfaction. And naturally a man wants to be a good lover and will proceed accordingly. **I also think the over-emphasis these days on oral sex reflects the reality that man has lost the art and the knowledge of how to use his penis and simply 'be present' in woman's vagina. He knows how to be excited, and how to ejaculate inside a woman's vagina, but just to be there in simple loving presence is a language yet to be discovered.** And equally woman needs to find out how to be receptive and relaxed, so that man can flower in her garden. **The focus on the clitoris definitely keeps man limited in his sexual horizons, not to mention woman herself.** So very little value is given to the penis *inside* the vagina and the result is that both men and women do not really know their true nature. Beautiful that you are so in touch with the intelligence of your body, and thank you!

Love, Diana

4. Thinking about intimacy and a lot of anger and disgust comes up

(The first part of this letter could be included in Chapter 3 on

Emotional Aspects, but because of its connection to the letter that follows on after it (below 5.), it has been placed in this chapter on Sexual Subjects.)

Dear Diana,

At the moment our love life is on ice and I would like to ask you for advice. In the last weeks I completely withdrew myself. There is no need or wish for intimacy. The good thing was that I experimented with listening inside myself. What really does nourish me in every moment? Because I notice that I am a master in manipulating myself to various concepts (also the concept to make love every day, even if it is perhaps necessary to be for my own for a few hours). But now several weeks have passed by and I also noticed that there is a collective anger against men in me. **I only have to *think* about intimacy and a lot of anger and disgust comes up. Anything I do against this resistance gives me the feeling I am manipulating myself.** Should I wait until there is a pull to meet each other again? But today I have the feeling there is no movement any longer in just waiting. It feels like a standstill. Perhaps you see other possibilities, and can give me advice on how we can approach each other again.

Love, Christine

Dear Christine,

The rage that is coming up in you is very real, and many women carry a deep sense of rage against men. **The source of this rage lies in sex. Not in sex per se, but what has happened to women in the name of sex. It can be due to the individual sexual past, and/or the female collective sexual rage and pain that lies accumulated in the past.** So basically the fact that your rage rises to the surface is very healthy because it is a layer stored inside your body and psyche that is coming up for cleansing and purification. Allowing this force through you will be empowering and integrating.

Most important is to realize that the anger is not against

your partner personally, but against the 'race' of man in general. A pretty girl will begin to encounter sexual looks and vibrations from men from a very early age, often with a tragic crossing of boundaries that can leave deep scars in her psyche. So women have good reason for the rage that gradually accumulates from childhood onward.

The most appropriate course of action is to allow the rage to flow out of you. Create a situation that invites the anger, and give way to its intensity. Best is to do this in private and apart from your partner. Go to a room, kneel on the bed/floor and beat a bunch of pillows with your fists, and without hurting yourself. Use the voice to shout or scream along with the beating, if you have a soundproof room. Continue for thirty or forty minutes, or for whatever amount of time is needed. Anger may turn into tears and sadness, with the feeling that you could cry for hours. Allowing the depth of this pain and sadness will cleanse your cells and your psyche.

You may wish to engage the assistance and support of a body therapist or breath therapist, someone who works in a body-oriented way. Moving your body on a regular daily level will also help substantially to discharge these emotions that build up. As soon as a layer of old emotion (unexpressed feeling) has moved out of your system then you will feel yourself quite differently, with a wish for intimacy and easily able to be in love.

Love, Diana

5. Different wishes regarding excitement and oral sex

Dear Diana,

Thank you for your answer (above 4.); it helped me to understand and accept what is going on. My partner was travelling for one week and there was a lot of time for myself alone. As he came back on Sunday, I suddenly felt so loving toward him. All anger was blown away and my heart opened wide. Unfortunately these lovely meetings end mostly in him trying to stimulate me. While accepting it, I feel that I close up in a way and lose this lovely connection to our hearts. After orgasm I feel miserable. He does not want to give up the stimulation. He would like to experiment with the stimulation while taking care of resting in our hearts. But for me that would be counterproductive. At the moment we have a different focus. I don't know how to arrange these different needs. It would not be a solution that he forces himself to cut off his longing for excitement.

So at the moment my partner's and my wishes appear to be moving in different directions, and I would like to ask for your advice. My wish for touch and stimulation of the clitoris in the last months has virtually disappeared. My partner really wishes that I touch and stroke his penis, and he also finds it frustrating that he cannot any longer stimulate me. But I feel no impulse, rather I have the feeling that touching of the genitals is very excitement fixated and I noticed it brings me out of the 'love energy'. He has the feeling that I ignore his penis, other than when we actually have sex. **I must admit that I feel very ambivalent toward the penis. Probably because earlier negative experiences and aggressive associations come to me quickly and I feel myself repulsed. When we do actually have sex together then it is different. Then I can focus on the energy and open myself.** How is it with kissing the genitals? Do you advise against it?

Love, Christine

Dear Christine,

There are really no rules to follow, and everything is fine, if it is done with awareness. It is always a matter of 'how' something is done, and not 'what' is done. When something is done with awareness it is naturally transformed through that very awareness. You have to explore and find new ways to do an old act. Sex, as we know it, is based on excitement so a person can easily remain oriented on that level of sensation because it is a pleasure. For some the intensity of excitement is addictive, and therefore not always easy to let go of. At the same time, relaxing away from the peaks of pleasure is a central point around which much personal exploration and experimentation is possible. This leads to tremendous transformation and growth.

I suggest that you trust your feeling not to have your genitals stimulated as is in traditional oral sex. It's not that oral sex is wrong, but it is more a question of it leading in the direction of excitement and discharging energy. Stimulating the clitoris can also lead to a lack of true sensitivity in the vagina. And, as you have already noticed, it can also cause a relative disturbance to the heart and love connection. This is a life-changing insight.

At the same time, it is nice that you do have genital touch rather than avoid it. Touch gently, with respect, and with the intention of increasing 'aliveness' instead of stimulating and causing excitement. **Learning to touch with awareness, warmth and presence is something quite different to stimulation. Conscious loving touch can help a person to bring their awareness more *inside* their genitals/body, and can enhance receptivity, sensitivity and sensuality.** It is so nice for a man when his woman warmly holds or lovingly caresses his penis. It is empowering as a man to feel his penis being valued and loved. So it is a matter of bringing the penis to life with love, rather than exciting it with erection or a climax in mind.

Many women will share your ambivalence about touching the penis, but this will change as you find ways of touching and making love that are not associated with stimulation and erection. Often what causes woman's ambivalence is the fear that when she touches him, he will get excited, get an erection, and will want to have sex then and there. And woman is often not prepared for that type of instant sex. Sometimes yes, but generally speaking she needs more time to warm up and open up.

I suggest that you start to touch the penis in a simple innocent way and support him in moving away from the conditioning/idea that genital touch equals stimulation and intensity. Equally a man needs to learn to touch the breasts of women with love and not stimulation. And to hold his cupped hand gently over the pubic mound area and send love. There is no need to stimulate the clitoris directly. The guideline is that touch should *expand* the energy of the person, help them to open up inwardly, feel themselves more deeply from within. On the other hand **excitement and intensity can make a person more extrovert, pulled to the periphery of experience/themselves. While a sensitive loving touch will make a person more introverted, connected to the inner** and encourage them to fall more deeply into their body.

I can understand your not wanting to ask your partner to change anything; but at the same time, it is your body in which love is made. And it's wise to honor its intelligence and your observations. Usually anything that is communicated to the partner, heart to heart, being to being, will be heard and honored. Speak about yourself and share your feelings. However be certain not to confuse them with your emotions where instead you end up speaking with some kind of 'charge' or tone of voice, and get into blaming, making him wrong, or saying things which are intended to hurt him.

The idea is to be loving and encouraging, and also to have compassion for man who has to step down from quite an exciting and stimulating program/conditioning. So in this sense woman does have to co-operate and encourage man and not alienate him. Be aware and loving in all you say and do. If a person is interested in personal growth, sex and love, then the way is to gradually transform sex from something dependent on excitement and goals, to something that is a relaxed experience of the here and now, the present moment. Time needs to be devoted to making love to create such a shift, and ultimately this inward turning is a spiritual search, a journey that will uplift and inspire your life in unforeseen ways.

Love, Diana

6. Helping erection to grow

Dear Diana,

Arriving home after the workshop with you so many thoughts were travelling through my mind. When you learn how to fly (I am a flying instructor) you start on a little training hill. At the end of the day, the talented pupils are maybe flying a little bit: for about a few seconds. The next day there is a very good chance that everyone gets this 'flying-feeling' and aims for more. Days with success and disappointment follow. On the fifth day, if the weather is good, a real flight is the highlight. Wow, feeling like a bird – looking all around. I have been flying for nineteen years. Not one flight has been like another. Flying in the high mountains of Pakistan and the deserts of Namibia, flying at our home in Germany. Now I know, flying is for me a path to my heart. The longer I fly, the more I can and want to learn about it. I think for me learning to make love in a new way will be much the same. How can I thank you for all your energy, your enthusiasm, your patience, and your love?

Now I have a question. When my man does a soft entry with an unerected penis – nothing happens. Should I start to move my pelvis from side to side, or should my man move back and forth. We noticed that when nothing happens the easiest but stupidest way is to fall back into the conditioned style. Please, tell us how we can help the penis to grow inside the vagina?

Love, Denise

Dear Denise,

The way you describe your experience of learning to fly is right on target as far as making love is concerned, thank you for that beautifully apt comparison. It is common, and to be expected, that 'nothing happens' when you initially do soft entry with an unerected penis. Like flying, you have to find your wings. And this requires time and practice. You need to start out with appreciating simple inner sensations, being accepting of whatever is, relaxing into the present and creating an environment of 'love' using your awareness. It is the presence of these qualities that gives the penis the capacity to extend in spontaneous erection. However this type of erection is definitely *not* something to be expected or wanted. In actual fact this type of internal erection happens when you are *not* thinking about it, when you are totally merged with your body and present to the moment. If you have a result in mind then you have a goal that puts you in the future, with the consequence that you are (in subtle ways and not so subtle ways) absent to the present.

Erection within the vagina most easily occurs when you get totally and utterly absorbed in the timeless present moment, feeling yourself deeply from the inside. Get your awareness into your vagina and create a welcoming receptivity within the tissues. And at the same time, and as a priority, connect inwardly with your breasts, and melt into them. This connects you with the female energy-raising pole, which brings you more deeply into polarity with the male force. This inner connection will for sure encourage and help to draw the penis, snakelike, into erection. Where there is expectation, not much is likely to happen.

Man's polarity is strengthened through being more and more present *in* his penis, and focusing on the perineum (lies just in front of the anus). Small movements as you are suggest are absolutely fine if it helps you to feel each other or encourage a bit of erection, but relax after a little while, and let the energy expand within your own bodies. And move again if you wish, and then relax. Anything you do with awareness naturally transforms through that awareness. Best wishes flying your inner and outer skies.

Love, Diana

7. I have completely lost my interest in sex

Dear Diana,

Well, I am a thirty-one year old male, in good health, got lots of energy and in love with life. I have had a fairly good sexual life with different lovers and partners, but recently I just don't feel like having sex at all. I have had a really lovely girlfriend for last six months. I am very expressive of lovingness with tactile embraces, hugs, cuddles, but when comes to sex it's just not there. I can get an erection, although sometimes not for long! I went to doctors and had medical check-up! My testosterone level is high apparently! I am not shy and nor do I feel that sex is bad! I feel a palpable loving feeling and passion for life! And my heart feels compassionate more than ever before!

In one way I feel calmer, collected and caring with everything in relationships of all kinds. In other way I feel for my girlfriend because she does want to have sex! Even though she expressed that she would love to have sex but she is fine going without it! I do feel honored and loved and really appreciated! I can see it in her eyes! I have suggested that if she wants to make love with other males, it's fine, but she is not into that. I want to hear from you. What is this? I am little bit confused! Am I impotent? Is my time up?

Love, Adrian

Dear Adrian,

It can happen that at a certain point in many people's lives that the efforts involved in conventional sex does cause sex to lose its charm, its pull, its attraction. This can be seen as part of a natural progression and unfolding of human sexuality, so rest assured, there is absolutely nothing wrong with you, and you are certainly not impotent, and for sure your time is not up! It is more a matter of knowing what the next step is, but unfortunately there is not really any alternative vision to guide us. And this leads to confusion and self-doubt, as you have experienced. To me what you are experiencing says very clearly that you are in touch with a deeper level of bodily awareness and intelligence, for which you can be grateful.

What is required is a complete revolution in the way you

think about and experience sex. In my books I have written a great deal of information and advice that will open doors for you, give you new sexual horizons that are inspiring. Usually sex involves a lot of tension and performance and goals, so the art lies in how to enter into sex in a relaxed and alive yet unexcited, unmotivated way. This is truly fulfilling and your interest in sex will be reawakened.

After reading any of my books I definitely suggest you try some things out with your girlfriend; choose a simple thing and put theory into action. Through personal experience you will come to know the deeper benefits of sex, and sex can become a guiding light your life.

Love, Diana

8. Pain in the testicles after not ejaculating

Dear Diana,

We are slowly starting to practice out of your book. For me it is very relaxing when my partner is inside of me, and doesn't move; then I can feel the energy expanding. When he starts moving, my body contracts and the energy field shrinks. We tried it a few times only without moving and were either too tired or couldn't continue because of the children, but every time my partner had an erection for some time and *didn't* ejaculate afterwards, he felt severe cramping pain in his testicles afterwards and felt very frustrated. So there are two needs opposing each other and we don't know how to continue. You mention in your book that men don't have to ejaculate necessarily, and my partner can't imagine how. Would you please give us any advice?

Love, Francesca

Dear Francesca,

Yes, we do say that men *do not have to ejaculate*; the point is that ejaculation has become a habit and it is valuable to explore other avenues. But *how* that non-ejaculation actually happens is significant. These pains after sex will usually come from one of two possible sources. One source of the pain is because the sex was more 'hot', building up energy, dancing on the verge of coming, and then *deliberately* this excitement/intensity has been repressed to avoid ejaculation. Basically here tension has been built up, and not discharged (as it usually is), so this can cause congestion and pain in the groin, penis, testicles, or lower belly afterwards.

For this reason we *do not recommend deliberate repression of ejaculation*. If a man finds himself on the verge of ejaculation, our suggestion is that he should ejaculate and not force himself to go against the tide.

However, it is essential to know that *pain can also be experienced afterwards when sex has been more 'cool'* and without the building up and repressing of excitement and tension. And this is what is confusing. In this second case the pain is positive and can be viewed as a 'healing pain', a reflection of old tensions/ memories leaving the body. The pains represent the cleansing and balancing of the genitals/whole system that takes place through having sex in awareness and relaxation.

In both cases, these pains will pass after some time, so there is nothing to be concerned about even though man is in physical discomfort. Having said this, if there is anything that is really worrying *please consult a doctor as soon as possible*.

A man in these painful circumstances will sometimes decide to masturbate in order to ejaculate the tension away. This is one solution, but doing so is again using and adding tension to an already tense congested situation. What is more beneficial is to get involved in some kind of gentle conscious body movement, shaking, dancing, walking, yoga or whatever, in order to support the pain to move out of the body.

Pains can very often also reflect unexpressed feelings, so it's good for a man to allow any feelings of sadness or insecurity (for example), that are coming to the surface through him.

As already mentioned, if a man finds himself very close to ejaculation it is really more appropriate to ejaculate right away, then and there. And not try to hold it down to prolong the sexual exchange, which is a tension. Repressing ejaculation involves tension so in the end a man is adding tension to tension which is in the long-term not a healthy situation.

So, if your man has pain you have to use the relaxation/ excitement or cool/hot guideline and ask yourselves, was sex more on the hot side or the cool side? And so you can monitor yourself and be in a better position to understand afterwards the source of any pain: Where there is pain after sex that was a bit hot/excitement zone, then the pain reflects tension accumulated in the body. But if there is pain after you have been cool in sex, then the pain is signifies tension being released. When tensions are dissolved in this second way it means that the genitals are relaxing and becoming more sensitive.

The general idea is to stay more present and cool in sex, to move away from sensation and toward sensitivity. But such a shift takes time and needs time. So it is quite natural that your partner cannot imagine how sex would look without ejaculation. The main thing is to make love for longer periods, and not to move straight toward ejaculation. It can be saved for two or three hours later. And when he does finally decide to ejaculate, then he can explore how he can do so in a more conscious relaxed way. This alone will enhance his experience. Just keep making love and through experimentation and exploration the focus and orientation will change over time. You begin to see sex in a different way.

Ejaculation itself is also okay; it's just that climax/orgasm has become the focus of sex, and usually the reason for having sex. When we change the focus and reasons for sex, then the view of ejaculation will also change. **There is certainly no rule to say that a man must not ejaculate, it is just the habit of having an ejaculation every time that is being questioned.** How would sex look (and how would I feel afterwards) if I contained the energy instead of discharging it - this time, instead of going with the habit again? It's a simple question and through enquiry it becomes possible to discover other realms and dimensions of sex.

Love, Diana

9. G-spot and female ejaculation

Dear Diana,

My partner and I started reading your book a few weeks ago. Even though intellectually I had not known some of the things you talk about, my body knew instantly and in reading your book I was 'reminded' of what I had always known in my body. It has been a most wonderful experience for my partner, and myself, and we are in fact recommending your book to all our friends whether or not they are in a relationship.

I am curious about one thing: you do not mention the 'G-spot' at all and you only mention the female ejaculate, 'amrita', once in passing. Other tantric schools put a lot of emphasis on this spot. Can you elaborate please?

Love, Gabriella

Dear Gabriella,

It is lovely to hear about your positive uplifting experiences with your partner, and the instant recognition of your essence is wonderful. In my view the G-spot is woven into a large tapestry of body tissues that are 'magnetically' sensitive and will encourage inner connections and streaming or movements of energy. There is no need to single out one point and make stimulating it some kind of a goal. Or likewise do not turn female ejaculation into a goal. **If contact happens between the penis and the G-spot naturally through the position for example, or if a woman ejaculates without effort, it is good. If these things do not happen of their own accord, then equally good. In fact, my whole approach is away from goals in the future toward presence, merging with your body in the here and now. And when truly connected on this level, all kinds of mysterious things can happen.** But they take place as an outcome or by-product of the level of presence, receptivity, relaxation and awareness.

It is possible that other tantra schools focus on these 'technical' aspects because they continue to approach sex from a conventional place, where sex has goals that involve doing something to get somewhere. My enquiry has been purely one from doing to non-doing, which is a fundamental level, and this exploration gives access to a vast inner cellular universe that in it is pure paradise. Another good reason for not pursuing the G-spot is that for woman her deepest orgasmic experiences are going to be due to a connection to her breasts and heart, thus melting into her positive energy raising pole, so why bother to get hooked up searching out the G-spot or trying to produce fluid? To me it makes no sense. Furthermore, woman is most receptive in the deepest part of her vagina (not the front where the G-spot is), and it is here she can tap into her divine energies.

A while ago I met a man who told me he had had two consecutive relationships where he had explored sex very deeply. The first woman did not ejaculate while the other ejaculated easily. When he got together with the second woman, he concluded that the difference must be because the first woman was somehow blocked, and not deeply open. However, after some years with the second woman, he realized that the sexual exchange with her was energetically *not* deeply moving or touching or transforming as it had been with the first woman. Even though the second woman ejaculated regularly. This observation points to the reality that it does not really matter whether the G-spot and/or ejaculation are experienced. He said that the first woman had a very loving welcoming heart and he sensed it was this aspect that made the qualitative difference to their sexual exchange. **So in my view additional goals are being set for woman that distract from her real essence, and there is no intrinsic value in running after them.** I hope my elaboration helps your under-standing.

Love, Diana

10. Techniques to build up energy

Dear Diana,

I am a man and I have been reading with great pleasure your book *Tantric Orgasm for Women* and it makes perfect sense to me. I would, however, appreciate some brief clarifications. Are you implying that there is little room for building up of energy? What I mean is, are there any circumstances where you'd recommend or allow for special pumping or rocking or breathing techniques as found in other approaches? You mention 'wild' sex. Is this possible without desensitization and contraction? Your responses to these questions would mean a great deal to me.

Thank you for your time and attention, I am glad I found you. On behalf of the planet, thank you for all that you do.

Love, Barry

Dear Barry,

Thank you for your writing. It is wonderful to hear that you as a man resonate with the book for women. The underlying question is always one of awareness. Whatever is done in and through awareness is transformed by that very awareness itself. There is a mysterious alchemy through which we can shift dimension. Awareness is a power, a force. **Tantra denies nothing but transforms everything, and the transformation happens through engaging awareness.** In that sense tantra is not a set of rules setting out what you can do and can't do, but it's an invitation to do whatever you enjoy, but to do so with heightened awareness. And that awareness itself is what makes the difference.

So for me it is not a question of what I do, but how I do it. My personal journey has been to shift away from goals and expectations, a journey from doing to being. Uncovering the intelligence of the body in the here and now. So in my picture the pumping etc. would represent doing with an outcome in mind. Certainly any of these techniques can be done as an occasional practice to intensify the connection to the body, but be sure to do them with awareness. There is a tendency to get mechanical and tense during any activity that is repeated again and again, so you will need to keep an eye on that.

The basis of technique involves making some kind of effort, and one day you will eventually need to relax from your efforts. And what then? To be more present to your body, just being and feeling what is going on with subtle energies present in the body. The inner polarity design is god given, it's always there, but inaccessible when we are busy doing.

As far as wildness is concerned, it's a matter for redefinition. What we know as 'wild' in sex is usually pretty unconscious, lust driven, tense and mechanical. So in this sense the experience is desensitizing because there is a tendency to contract at a deep level, and there will be no room for expansion. **As I understand and experience it, lust and passion are two different states. Lust will have a direction, a build-up, some climax. Passion on the other hand is pure presence and going nowhere, relaxed, senses totally open, nothing forced.** True 'wildness' is to be at one with nature, utterly sensitive and conscious, opening to the moment through the body. Wildness has no pattern, the bodies spontaneously flow and form amazing configurations.

So the art is to do whatever you do with awareness, and to explore sex through this window. In general, the idea is to transform one's inherited conditioning that is sensation and orgasm driven, to a style where you anchor yourself in the here and now, no objective in mind, and create the situation for sensitivity and ecstasy.

Love, Diana

11. Balancing negative effects of peak orgasm

Dear Diana,

Thank you so much for your reply (above 10.) Yes, okay I understand now, anything goes if we're conscious, and that discovering how to be present in itself will help overcome our drive-to-orgasm conditioning. I have one last question. I gather a number of students engage in conventional sex for a while alongside of tantric lovemaking. If immediately after conventional sex I keep the penis inside the vagina, and with deep awareness, does this avoid the negative consequences of peak orgasm sex? Has anyone noticed whether connecting the genitals and being aware right after conventional sex helps to mitigate some of the consequences like energy drain, emotional build-up, etc.? Or for couples who, in your words, entertain desire a few seconds too long while trying to be conscious and get swept up to a peak, does relaxing, plugging in and deepening awareness at that point, after orgasm, help counteract some of the energy drain and emotional build-up? I suppose these questions are one in the same.

Another last question. Years ago I had a series of kundalini up the spine experiences without technique, unexpected. Are you and your students finding the same? That is by just being and being led by inner wisdom without special sacred techniques that these risings and cosmic awareness happen? Or should some chakra visualization and energy cultivation be done beforehand?

Love, Barry

Dear Barry,

Regarding your first question, yes, certainly lying together after climax/orgasm is going to be helpful, in that you have time to unite on the level of the being. And it will help to avoid emotional reactions that can happen after energy has been discharged. **Women often feel feelings of abandonment, loneliness, or sadness. Men tend to lose interest, disconnect and turn away once they have spent their energy, so taking the time to unite is very restoring. But the energy is wasted nonetheless.** And the opportunity to see what else could have happened has passed.

As to your second question, very definitely spontaneous energy happenings can occur in the body, without specific preparation or using a special technique. And it is beautiful that you have had these experiences spontaneously. Visualization can be a help but not essential, as you discovered. Imagining light, or gold, or streaming can ignite or prompt inner energy movements, at the same time visualization then easily becomes a focus for the attention and a subtle form of inactive 'doing'. Through this, a slight, yet significant, element of 'simply being' is lost. So on one level visualization helps; on another level it does not help! You have to experiment with it. The miracle is that energy does follow imagination, so visualization can be a powerful tool at times. (And we know that this is true because of sexual fantasy often used in conventional sex – it works!)

The kind of energy cultivation that I would recommend beforehand would be for you as man to begin to root your awareness in your perineum, the male positive pole, something quite simple. You do so during your daily activities, not only when you are in bed. And generally, you can cultivate your energy level by doing some exercises that you enjoy. Choose anything that helps you to direct and root your attention to the subtle inner realms of your body.

Love, Diana

12. I have never had an orgasm

Dear Diana,

Since meeting you in a workshop, I now have a new man in my life. I connected with an old friend who I had not seen for seven years. And we fell in love and are together since. I guess you'll find us in The Making Love Retreat some time. It's wonderful to be with him, and we match sexually really well, although we connect in a normal (conventional) way, and not so much in the way I learned and experienced in your workshop with my previous partner. And still it's fulfilling. **What I experience is that I still cannot have an orgasm or I don't know how it feels to have one. I have lived with that my whole life.** And sometimes it makes me sad; I think being orgasmic must be wonderful. And me not having an orgasm gives also some kind of stress in the relationship with my man. He sometimes thinks he's not good enough – although I talk to him openly. Somehow I have given up having an orgasm and still there is this little flame burning – why not me also?

Love, Irene

Dear Irene,

I am really pleased to hear that you have met an old friend who is now your lover. The orgasm issue is a delicate subject, but in the end it is how you view the whole theme that will make the difference. In usual sex, orgasm is the goal and often the reason for sex; while in tantra there is no interest or value given to building up the energy to a peak or climax. **So, this means that in the conventional sense you do have a problem, and in the tantric sense *you do not have a problem*.** It just depends on you how you deal with it! What I can say without a shadow of doubt is that there is nothing wrong with you because you did not manage a conventional orgasm. **You are in company with millions of women. Usually conventional orgasm is due to a build-up of tension or excitement that takes effort and focus or fantasy.** Rarely do orgasms occur through simply doing nothing. If you are not managing an orgasm then I can say everything is really perfect as it is! It means that your whole system and senses are geared toward sensitivity and relaxation, your body does not respond to pressure, tension and effort.

Now you are undermining yourself with thoughts about how you have never had an orgasm. Instead you can use that same energy and invest it in your awareness, and go for relaxation, sensitivity, and expansion. Develop an interest in your inner cosmos, the intercellular life and pleasure that exists on a very subtle level. It is here that you will be able to tap into the source of orgasmic or ecstatic experiences. So in this sense there is a big difference between having a conventional orgasm, and being truly orgasmic. And far as higher orgasmic experiences are concerned, firstly these will not and *do not happen every time* you make love. And secondly, when they do arise there will be a deep melting connection to the breasts and heart. **You will remember that in tantra the breasts are the key to accessing and awakening the female sexual energy, and not the vagina or clitoris.**

So you can begin to bring your breasts and nipples into the foreground of your awareness as you make love. Not in a tense focused way, but in a melting merging inner way. You can also gently cup and hold your own breasts. A woman can do much to influence the situation in positive ways through awareness and receptivity. And there is much you can do independently of your partner. Even though he does not consciously know about the tantric approach, your presence and relaxation is going to touch him in invisible and mysterious ways.

Love, Diana

13. Pulsating, hot, wonderful breasts, my own power plant

Dear Diana,

This morning I want you to be the first person I write to. I am so deeply touched and happy! I am lying on my bed with my computer on my knees. I am here with pulsating, hot, wonderful breasts and it does not stop! As if I had my own power plant. For the first time I feel what it really means to 'be' a woman. **I finally understand what you always keep saying: remember your positive poles, your breasts - it is really good!** I stand before the mirror and I hold my breasts and I 'am'. An incredible energy, I get hot and I radiate! I feel that this really is my place of creativity. I am awake and everything I do, I do it 'through' my breasts. It started in the group with you that I perceived my breasts both hot and pulsating. Now it continues!

During the group I decided to always 'receive' my partner, no matter what I 'feel like'. When we arrived back home yesterday evening it was very emotional and I feared our new appointment would not happen. But I remembered my promise, talked to my partner, and we met anyway. He did the some exercises and I searched for my polarity and then we had a short tantric exchange. First I felt the time pressure but still I held my breasts and made contact with them. **Even when my partner fell asleep I stayed with myself and then suddenly I could feel them pulsating and the penis grew inside of me. It was wonderful.**

When we subsequently separated I insisted that we separate consciously, and I told him that I could still feel him even though he was not inside me anymore. Then I stood in the hallway and my breasts radiated and pulsated and they still do. I feel like being in love and above all now I know 'who' I am.

Being here feels completely different. Now, after being with you in a few groups, I know that I have responsibility for myself and that I really only have to come to myself, in my breast pole and everything changes – my feeling for myself and my beloved, for the day and in general. **I am connected to my breasts as I write. And I understand why it is so important to look into the world inside. The soft vision that takes me inside, simply being in the world. Just now I feel this state of being and it really changes everything.**

I am so thankful and so happy that I kept on going and did not give up even though I often felt like it, not finding my way in the dark. Now I have it inside of me, now I know who I am in my soul. The dark has disappeared via light, just as Osho describes it. I feel this new quality. And I am sure it is also connected to our decision to trust love instead of fear. I have tears in my eyes and I send you a warm hug!

Love, Samantha

Dear Samantha,

Thank you so much for sharing your life-changing breast experiences, and it is especially touching because of the challenging moments you have had along the way. It is very significant that you have observed what a big shift takes place when you come home to yourself, where there is less worrying about what the other is doing or is not doing. It is a lesson for us all! I am so happy for you and I appreciate your sincerity and searching. Discovering that you can so easily make the difference is one of the greatest revelations. Best wishes to you both.

Love, Diana

14. I asked my lover to withdraw his penis a fraction

Dear Diana,

My lover described the experience today as we faced each other in one of the positions that allow deep penetration (him, kneeling; me, lying down) as 'alive' and the sensations as 'so soft' and 'so subtle'. Today I seemed to have little sensation, not sexual and not the tingly, blissful sensations of energy either. I became aware of tension in my mind and body and used your method of the 'turning in and looking/scanning' to relax the body tensions. As I did so, I became more and more relaxed until my mind state changed. It was as if I fell off the edge of the known universe, just a very relaxed space of being. Hard to describe. Very open, very relaxed, gone... but I could still talk.

I put together later what happened after the change in my mind state. As you suggest when there is some kind of pain in the vagina, I asked my lover to withdraw his penis just a hair/fraction because of an odd sensation, this time like an eyelash in the eye. He did this and the energy on the left side of my pelvic bowl expanded exponentially, surprising me and making me laugh heartily. He began to laugh because I was laughing – and that ended the physical connection. You do mention that laughter or tears as a form of cleansing/releasing tension are not unusual in this process.

We rested for a while, held each other, and talked and then moved into the scissors side position. The same spot in my vagina that had expanded began to ache and I put my hand over it or asked him put his hand there. At the end we did not move at all for a long time. He whispered, "My penis is caressing you."

Then, it seemed as if his penis were scanning my body. It shined a light first over the right side of the body then the left. I imagine it was energy that I was experiencing but I 'saw' it as light. The light was unobstructed and sparkly throughout my body except in the spot on the left side of the pelvic basin. There it looked different, more like a shadow on an X-ray. I was moved to say to him, "Your penis loves me." His penis also seems very wise.

Love, Sasha

15. Advice for our tantric exploration

Dear Diana,

We have been making love much more often since we have been to your retreat, which could not have been imagined earlier. I would like to ask for your advice: when my husband is in me (in the side position) without any or only very, very little movement, it is very nice for me. I can relax and breathe and expand and feel touched somewhere deeper in me. For my husband it is somehow nice, too, and also it easily becomes a little bit boring for him and sometimes he falls asleep. Thus he tends to move more, preferring to lie on top of me. With this it is very hard for me not to get excited, either I have a (down regulated) orgasm or I feel charged especially in the area of the clitoris (which does not feel comfortable).

If I discharge by the usual orgastic contractions of the vagina, afterwards it takes some time to find my way back to sensitivity and the feeling of being connected to my husband (actually this small orgasm thing for me feels somehow like an abuse of the given opportunities of sexual energy). Is there a way to keep cool with his movement or should I ask him to regulate it down even more? Or do you have any other suggestion?

This tantra stuff really is difficult and easy at the same time. It is a process of 'fighting' against excitement, and at the same

time experiencing 'states' that we could never reach by ourselves through making effort. I consider it a very precious gift to feel my husband in such a beautiful male dynamic energy (which has been twice so far). There is a very rare feeling comes up in me: I deeply admire him in this 'state' and it feels so good to feel like that.

Then it feels even worse the other times when we are not present enough, when excitement is coming up instead! Then I need to remember those real wonderful situations to get the courage to try again. Your retreat was one of the most precious gifts I ever received in my life. Thank you so much for that!

Love, Kathrin

Dear Kathrin,

I am really pleased to hear that you are making love regularly in the months since the group. It does happen that a woman is happy with the simplicity, less effort and being less active. While for the man, because there is not much feeling there is the wish for some movement to increase the intensity and sensation. This wish or need is very real because of how man has learned to have sex. To 'do' and build up intensity is part of the male conditioning in sex. In the absence of sensation it is quite normal not to 'feel', not to have much inner perception and sensitivity. And then boredom can set in.

On one hand this aspect (conditioning around sensation) must be respected, integrated. So it is good if you accept his movement, but you can ask for conscious movement, not mechanical movement. This will also increase *his* sensitivity, the capacity to feel. I suggest you don't 'join in' with his movement, let him move, and you focus on relaxing the vagina, receiving the penis, connecting with your breasts. In this way you can stay cool, and you will also cool him down.

And on the other hand the conditioning must also be challenged, in order to transform the pattern and conditioning and habit so that something new is able to evolve. Energetic openness of woman is basic to a deeper flow of energy and love between man and woman, so her inner expansion is somewhat of a priority. If woman's body is open something is possible, when her body is closed, not much is possible. Clitoral stimulation can play a part in a woman's body/vagina closing. The vagina gets excited but this is a very different environment to one of receptivity. **And yes, you have noticed yourself how the vagina loses sensitivity when the clitoris is engaged.** Excitement/orgasm in conventional sex usually happens through a build-up of tension, so ultimately it is a type of contraction, and not an expansion. (Unless getting to a climax is 'managed' very consciously through relaxation.) So perhaps it's good for you to avoid a situation where your clitoris get stimulated, and stay true to what opens you, what expands your body energy, what touches your heart.

The guideline is 'it's not what you do but how you do it', so there are no rules like you must *not* have an orgasm or quit moving. Anything done with awareness is transformed by that awareness, so if you decide to have an orgasm, see how relaxed you can be in it, how easy, connected, and present. Already this changes the experience dramatically. If you feel like moving during sex, try undulating cat-like stretches that engage the fascia (connective tissue), and help energy to move through your body.

Try some variations in position to keep your husband more awake. A bit of sleeping now and then while making love is also very nice and a form of deep relaxation. And even if one sleeps the other can stay connected to his/her own inner world. The deep and overwhelming urge to sleep, the eyes closing without be able to control it, can sometimes be a sign or indicator of feelings hiding beneath the surface, so it's good for him to check that out. Great if he (and you) can get a massage every week, and both do some exercise immediately before entering bed, or have a shower to freshen up. Energizing yourself before making love is a great support.

Another possibility, which can be very helpful, is to *not* think about this genital meeting as 'sex'. Instead, think of it as a simple union, a meditation, a deep relaxation, and a subtle bonding of energy fields. When we think of the meeting as 'sex' then comparisons and expectations come in, which naturally lead to boredom because something is not happening. If we don't have these expectations, and we know what we are in for, it is much easier to relax and accept what 'is', and to 'be' in the body. If you both change your 'minds' then it is easy to let this style of union unfold with practice and patience. **And then notice how you feel afterwards, within yourself and between you. In this way afterwards is always your teacher. The orientation of tantra is to reach to the being and the source of love lying within**.

Love, Diana

Dear Diana,

Thank you for your helpful reply. Last night I was really frustrated and sad. It had been difficult to keep this date set for yesterday, because my husband is on a business trip today and tomorrow, Thursday and Friday I have to attend school meetings. Thus I ironed his clothes and asked him for an evening date again. And he was there in time and he was not sleepy at all. His penis was erect even before entering me.

I guess I was slightly 'emotional' that afternoon, not knowing the reason why. And when we came together I felt very open and very sensitive and it took only a few minutes for me to 'come' with almost no stimulation; I had no chance to keep it down and then I felt distant from my partner, sad, frustrated, couldn't feel him anymore, and wished I were miles away. Where is the point?

Love, Kathrin

Dear Kathrin,

Sometimes the excitement will just be there, in one person or the other person or both. But in time with frequency of lovemaking, as you are doing, this superficial level of excitement reaction will reduce, because sex becomes more normal and natural. Usually when excitement in a woman gets to a high level as she builds up to a climax, then old tensions will be discharged down the vagina, which can easily have the effect of making a man ejaculate instantly. These old tensions in woman's body also reduce in time, especially with the deep sustained penetration, which we suggested during the retreat.

The tensions of emotion can also be the cause/source of excitement and, as you were aware, you were already a bit emotional from the afternoon. So then you had an orgasm and felt disconnected afterward. This is very interesting. No need to judge, but simply to observe and learn how all these things are connected in subtle, or not so subtle ways. You are an intelligent person, with profound insights, so keep a distance to these happenings, be more of an observer, and remember a sense of humor is a good friend. I learned in the same way – by trial and error as we say in English.

I feel that you are doing extremely well, going about it in a scientific way, learning through practice and using afterwards as your teacher. It is so interesting to observe the two different states, and great that you experience them so clearly. Through having this experience again and again you will fall away from the excitement habit gradually and naturally. Or when excitement arises and you feel yourself starting to follow through to a climax then start to investigate how you can do that more easy, more relaxed, with as little 'doing' as possible, staying more in your being, using tantric principles at the same time, even as you go for orgasm. Actually, relaxation improves the experience of conventional orgasm too.

Basically, you are on a slow process of deconditioning yourself and it takes time and you need patience, sense of humor, willingness to keep taking steps forward. I appreciate the reminder contained in Osho's words "... life is a mystery to be lived and not a problem to be solved..."

Love, Diana

Dear Diana,

Thanks a lot for your mail, your listening and understanding and advice.

You give me hope and courage to go on. Your heartful accompaniment and supervision helps me so much! With deep thankfulness and best wishes to you and Michael.

Love, Kathrin

16. Combining tantric sex with conventional sex

Dear Diana,

There is something that I have wanted to ask you for some time because it is an area of confusion for me. I have done a few groups with you now and you tell us very clearly not to make a separation between the 'new' way and the 'old' way. I have heard that some teachers of tantra are telling people to do conventional sex and tantric sex parallel with each other. By this is meant that sometimes they do it one way, and at other times they do it another way. What is your opinion about this type of separation?

Love, Laura

Dear Laura,

Thank you for writing – it is a good question! In the field there seems to exist a deep misunderstanding that is based on lack of personal experience. The basic problem is that people make a separation between one and the other where in reality no separation exists. Tantra is not a technique – not something that you 'do' – rather it is a process of becoming more conscious through shining the light of awareness on the sex act. In tantra we are transforming an unconscious force into a conscious force. So in essence, we need to start introducing awareness into sex – that is all. And we have to start from where we are – which is conditioned in a certain style of sex that has become the convention.

You start to observe yourself not *what* is done, but *how* it is done. And gradually the sex energy is transformed into a meditative energy through this enquiry. It is impossible to drop the conditioning overnight because the patterns are deeply lodged in our psyche and cells. So in that sense there will naturally be a floating between how you have done it in the past and the new track that you are exploring. In time the more conscious style takes root and overturns the conventional patterns. So to me there is no question of doing it conventional one time, and tantric the next time.

Basically this suggests that tantra is something you do as a special technique from time to time – like lie without moving inside each other for some hours – this does not make any sense at all.

The endeavor and the adventure should be to enter into sex with as much awareness as you can, every time you make love! Not only sometimes. Conventional sex is based more on sensation, and tantric sex more on sensitivity. How can you grow in sensitivity if you continue to support sensation? Sensation kills sensitivity, so you will go around in circles. In the morning asking your genitals to be sensitive and then in the night asking them to be sensational. There should be no separation. We are conditioned to be hot and excitement based, so the journey is to transform this pattern slowly, to become cooler and more sensitive. **It is only in a cool relaxed environment that the deeper potential of sex can manifest itself in the timeless experiences of bliss and ecstasy.**

It is a process of deconditioning yourself – rooting out the habits and patterns that dominate sexual expression. Once you are free of these tensions, then you will always make love in a different way – with more awareness and presence. Sometimes participants in our groups will ask if we (my partner and I) ever have hot sex 'now and then'? But again such a question reflects the same misunderstanding. Once you are conscious in sex it is extremely difficult to be unconscious in sex! How to be sensitive one time and insensitive the next? Every time you have sex in the future, it will be transformed by that awareness. If you chose to move, the movements will not be mechanical and goal oriented, but relaxed and easy, each move pure pleasure unto itself. Or if you choose to have an orgasm you will do so in a way that expands the body energy rather than contracts and localizes it in the genitals.

Osho says very simply:"Tantra is the transformation of sex into love through the awareness," and I always find these words to be tremendously inspiring. I hope my explanation has helped to sort out your very understandable confusion in this area.

Love, Diana

Chapter 5

Special Issues

1. Healing the physical pains in my vagina

Dear Diana,

When I heard the audiotapes of Barry Long about making love for the first time, maybe ten years ago, it changed my way of looking at sexuality completely. Everything I vaguely was feeling in myself, he was acknowledging. But there remained a lot of practical questions. In my lovemaking, I experienced more and more great physical pain, which finally made lovemaking impossible. I went to a lot of gynecologists and they told me I had focal vulvitis or vaginitus or vulvodynia, nobody really knew. The years that followed, I tried everything to heal the state of my vagina and slowly, slowly things got better. But the pain still was there a lot of the time and I really was thinking I was crazy and getting really worried if I ever would be able to make love again. The thing I loved doing most. I moved into a new relationship where making love was still not possible in the beginning. Then I got hold of your book *The Heart of Tantric Sex*. I did quite some reading and experimenting in other tantric versions, but for me it always felt to be unnatural in some sort of way. With your book, I felt I was coming home. I was so happy to read in your book about the female side of making love in which everything was resonating with my inner feeling of what making love was all about. And then I read your second book *Tantric Orgasm for Women* and that was all I ever have wanted to know since I was young. Thank you very much for sharing all your wisdom with me, I feel so grateful for it. Especially with all the other women's sharing's in the book and also your comments about pain, I now for the first time see how my pain might have been started and how it possibly can be reversed itself - by making love with a loving penis. I would have never thought that the penis, the actual thing that hurt my vagina, could make it better again. And then my partner read the book too, so we changed our way of lovemaking and then I was more open and I could receive his penis. And when the pain was there, we could stop and wait and then slowly continue. After a while I was open again and we could make love several times without pain. I was ecstatic. And I know now that it might be possible to heal completely for I know the pain is not gone completely. But I feel now a confidence in me I never felt before.

Since my partner lives in another country, I think I need to work on my own a lot and I might need some massage of my vagina. In your book you talk about massaging the vagina. You mention it in one sentence. Could you please tell me a little bit more about it? What more do you know about vaginitis/vocal vulvitis or vulvodynia and do you know any woman that healed from it completely? For years I looked for one woman, who could inspire me, by showing me she did it. No woman was there, but I keep hoping I will find her and maybe I will be that woman.

Love, Zoe

Dear Zoe,

Thank you for your e-mail and I am pleased to hear that you and your partner have had some positive and encouraging experiences through applying the information in my books. My feeling and experience is that this style of making love will be ultimately healing. The fact that you have had pain-free sex a few times is a good indicator. And it shows you that relaxation and awareness is the right path to follow. And yes, it is a relief and inspiration to realize that the penis has great healing power when used consciously. I had contact some years ago with a Brazilian organization that dealt with these female issues of vaginal pain, and they were having good results using the suggestions in my book. In my courses I have met many women who had an issue around painful penetration, and definitely the slow conscious style of sex makes pain-free penetration possible.

Yes, I do mention massage of the vagina briefly; but in truth, if you have a loving man in your life then the penis is the best way to go. It is not so easy to find a person to do this type of massage, and for many years now I have not used it for myself or suggested it to others. Mainly because in reality the fingertip is quite rough in relation to the very sensitive fine vaginal tissues, plus the finger is not really designed for that place or piece of work. Whereas the head of the penis is like a highly sensitive magnet, and this grants it an innate intelligence that speaks directly to the vagina.

So I feel it's best that you relax with what is. I also suggest that you do not masturbate (if you are doing so) because you are in subtle and unsubtle ways adding tensions to an already fragile and tender situation.

And you will certainly benefit from meditating on your breasts and bringing awareness to the female positive pole. Doing so on a daily basis (for about a half hour) will naturally have some healing resonance in the vagina. My partner and I have published a guided meditation on the breasts especially for women called *MaLua Light Meditation*. The music and voice may support you to go deeper into yourself. Let me know how you get along.

Love, Diana

Dear Diana,

Thank you so much for your response. Your answer came just at the right time. Between the mail I wrote to you and your answer back, I, for the first time, discovered a website about vulvodynia, with a few women who talk about their recovery. One recovered with natural hormones and a few because they had an over activity of the nerves in the labia and opening of the vagina. They were operated on and then they could have normal sex again. After I read that, I was extremely happy and I looked really deep into that website, and a whole world opened up, about other doctors having written books about the subject, which I never had seen before.

But soon I realized that I got so confused and stressed by it, that, I think, the pain in my vagina got worse again. It made me realize that by reading about all the women who were in pain, or not, my thinking about it, and so my body was affected in a negative way. I came into that painful energy of wanting results; instead of that energy I was in, when reading your book, the energy of beauty, female essence and strength. All I could do was leave the subject aside and only try things like the natural hormones, or some kind of calcium for a better nerve activity.

What I realized vaguely was that almost none of the women I read about were talking about *the way they practiced sex*, that it could be a cause for their pain, or that a loving penis could be the healer. But I had, in a way, also forgotten about it, in all the confusion the information caused in me. But when I read your response, you directly lead me to that truth inside of me – that truth of being rather than to put the accent on the doing part.

Everything you write makes me feel that this is what I want to do and it all feels so natural. I hope to find myself a nice man, who lives closer, and one who really wants to get to know, or already knows, the way of lovemaking you are teaching. The reason is that I have decided to split up with my American lover, although the lovemaking was beautiful. I have a dream of having that kind of lovemaking on a more regular basis, than just once and awhile, so my vagina can truly heal. In between that time I will order the *MaLua* CD and practice the breast meditation, which I think will indeed be of support. Thank you again for your sweet words.

Love, Zoe

Dear Diana,

Hello again and here is an update! Things are indeed evolving in very good way since I last wrote to you. **I stopped doing all the things I thought I needed to do**, like taoistic energy exercises, with or without jade egg, circulating the energy around in my body and masturbating. **All these things made me stressed out, somehow. I think because these things I did were all based on fear, and the belief that something was terribly wrong with me.** And that if I didn't do them then my hormones wouldn't get better, or the bloodstream wouldn't be optimized, so that my vagina would never heal. It was also a way to check to see if I finally could enter my vagina, for instance, with my finger or a little tube or egg, in order to get my vagina used to the entering of a penis. But the last time I actually had intercourse without pain, made me realize that a loving penis would be the best way to heal my vagina and that all the other ways seemed only to get in the way of that belief. In that loving way, I could finally surrender to beauty and love, instead of giving in to fear and anxiety.

Since a loving penis is at the moment not within reach, I have had to create that loving environment in myself. So I did what you suggested and it was what I always thought somewhere deep down would be the best, but I never trusted myself, for it seemed too easy. I started to lie down more often and especially when I had pain. Just doing nothing and feeling, relaxing, and enjoying. In all that, energy begins arising, I feel my breasts and feel also what a sensuous and lively woman I am. This gives me such an amount of peace.

For a long, long time, I always had thought of myself as not being a real woman, because I couldn't have painless sex. I felt totally inadequate as a woman and I felt a strong need to make love to a man in order to feel as a woman. But now there is this sense of female beauty, and I feel that I am no longer dependant on anything else, or a man who penetrates me. Of course I love to be penetrated in a loving way, but I see that there is such beauty in me beyond that, and that always will be available for me at any time, or any place.

The only thing I tried was to use a natural progesterone cream. This seems to help tremendously. The pain is now only sometimes there and I have good hopes it will be gone completely somewhere in time. All these wonderful developments even made me think that I want to share this beauty with other women and become what I always wanted to find when I was so desperate: to be a woman who has healed and can inspire other woman in doing that too!

Love, Zoe

2. How to get pregnant when there is reduced ejaculation?

Dear Diana,
A few months ago I read your books and my husband and I are

very happy with our new experiences of making love. Thank you! We both want to have a baby and so I want to ask you if there is perhaps a tantric way of making love with a baby wish? How to get pregnant when there is reduced ejaculation? Can you recommend any books about this theme? Thank you for your inspiration!

Love, Yvette

Dear Yvette,

Thank you for writing. I am delighted to hear that you are having valuable experiences through experimenting in love, and my congratulations — all credit goes to the two of you because you are doing it for yourselves, not just reading about it. It's really one of those things that have to be tried out to know the truth and value of it.

Regarding having a baby, I cannot point you toward any books that I know of but I must say that I have not researched this field. I feel the most important thing is to realize that basically the way things stand almost all conception happens in an accidental way. A couple wants to have a child, but the invitation is general and not specific, very seldom is the moment for conception (ejaculation) consciously planned and followed through on.

Most people, if you ask them (which I do in my groups), will say that subjectively they felt abandoned at some level, and did not feel truly welcomed and wanted by their parents. **So one great step you can make is to ensure that conception is conscious, and that takes place in great love and with intention.** Practically this means to find out when you are most fertile through the temperature method/quality of mucous discharge etc., and then go for the conception on the right day/s.

Create a beautiful atmosphere for the occasion, and prepare your bodies too, bathing, dancing or anything 'physical' to bring you into your body energies.

Now the interesting point is the following, based on something that I have heard Barry Long say, that ejaculation should ideally take place as soon as possible after entry. And it is recommended that the woman does *not* have or try to have an orgasm at the same time. For actual conception purposes the more simple the act the better. A pure simple authentic act can be done with great love and awareness, preparing yourselves and the space around you as an invitation to creation. May your wishes to have a family be fulfilled in an effortless and joyful way.

Love, Diana

3. Absence of breasts due to surgery

Dear Diana,

I have just found your book and am beginning to read all the information you provide there. It is difficult for me to deal with the input on breasts because I lost my breasts because of cancer a few years ago. I felt so much pain and sorrow at the loss of femininity that I have avoided sex since then. I am finally beginning to heal and open to love again, but I really feel the absence of my breasts. I am just learning about tantra. What of my situation?

Love, Wanda

Dear Wanda,

My heartfelt condolences to you on your tremendous loss and I send you much love and healing energy. Yes, in the tantric view, the breasts are the place where energy is raised in the female body. On the surface this makes the approach difficult for you, and I can appreciate your feelings. **What is interesting and very encouraging, however, is that the intrinsic energy-raising capacity in the breasts is an energetic phenomenon and not something purely physical.** I did not know this for a fact at first, but over the years I have had several women in my courses, in a similar situation to yours, and each one said that they could feel the 'energetic response' or 'energetic overflow' of the breasts in the vagina, even in the absence of the physical breasts. So in this deeper sense your energy centers are intact and continue to function perfectly. Please read my second book called *Tantric Orgasm for Women* where breasts as an aspect of femininity is covered in more detail.

It would also be very healing if you begin to meditate on your chest and heart area for about twenty minutes a day, holding your hands gently over the chest, and melting into and merging with your heart. Doing breast meditations regularly will support in reconnecting with your feminine qualities, even if there are no physical breasts. You may be interested in getting the MaLua guided breast meditation with music (CD) produced by my partner and myself. I know there is nothing that can ever replace what you have lost, but in the meantime the tantric information gives you a positive view that will give you the strength and capacity to move forward in an enriching way. Best wishes to you.

Love, Diana

4. No information on the chakra system

Dear Diana,

I'm right now reading your book *The Heart of Tantric Sex* that I feel very inspired by. My girlfriend is reading *Tantric Orgasm for Women*. She's very inspired and I was very curious when she got the book. I heard that you are doing a book for men and I'm really looking forward to reading it. Will you say something about healing the penis? I've been exploring tantra and Taoism for about eighteen months. A few months ago I participated with my partner in a tantra course in Sweden that was a wonderful, loving and painful experience due to old emotional wounds. That's where I got the information on your books.

During that course, they talked about the different polarities of the seven chakras. When I read your book you focus on the first and fourth chakras, and there is no mention polarities of the other chakras. Or have I missed something? During the course I attended they focused a lot on the male's first and the female's second chakra. I was really curious to learn more about polarities and the parts that are described in your books were useful but I hoped to find more information in your books on all chakras. I'd like to know why you chose not to mention them in the books?

Love, Xavier

Dear Xavier,

Yes, you are right, there is virtually no information about the chakras (energy centers), and this is with intention. I personally was never able to connect with any objective information I read or heard about the chakras – it did not speak to me. So in this sense information on the chakras was not a part of my sexual exploration. And therefore I do not give them much attention in my books. I don't even really think about my chakras ever; they are alive and active and doing their thing whether I know about them or think about them. At times my chakras show themselves through inner energy experiences, but these are subjective experiences and more the outcome of having made love in a certain way for a while.

My experience and understanding of sex is more as a 'magnetic flow' that arises through the existence of opposite poles in the body. The sex center being the one pole and the heart center the second. This is the reason for my referring to these two chakras only. As I said already, chakras are present and functioning in your body whether you know about them or not. You have simply to set the stage and the inner workings happen in their own time and in their own way. Certainly what I discovered was that through aligning my sexual behavior according to our 'magnetic' design, many notable experiences in all my seven chakras took place. But these happened as by-products of my explorations, not due to any intention or due to any information about the chakras.

So my focus in teaching/writing is to explain the basic set-up and encourage people to explore, get the bodies polarized and 'magnetically aligned', and then see what happens. Too much information can give readers an excess of food for thought that eventually gets in the way as expectations and goals, and a person gets waylaid and loses touch with more essential elements of tantra.

The book for men will be called *Tantric Sex for Men* and will include penis healing and balancing, which according to my approach happens through focusing on the perineum to ground your male energy and being conscious and present inside the female vagina.

I wish you all the best in your exploration, and trust that you will find my books useful, even without the chakra information that you were hoping for!

Love, Diana

5. Can tantra have a therapeutic influence on massage?

Dear Diana,

I am doing massage and want to know how tantra can be used to influence my massage in a therapeutic way? There is a lot of tantric massage around that involves touching the genitals but I am not interested in that.

Love, Lucy

Dear Lucy,

During a massage I would suggest that you start including tantric principles, which in essence means you must relax and be aware as you massage. I was a massage teacher for 20 years, and in retrospect I have realized that massage was in fact the start of my tantric journey, exploring the inner world of my own body. So as a giver of massage you are in a very good situation to begin encountering yourself and your own body in a new way. You will find the instructional massage DVD, called *Time for Touch - Massage, Awareness, Relaxation,* a great help in learning tantric massage.

Tantra basically implies a turning inward or introversion, so it is my suggestion that you make yourself and your body the center of the enquiry and not the other person who is receiving the massage. I know it sounds odd! It will help you to read *The Heart of Tantric Sex,* where I list and describe the 'love keys', and start to introduce these into your massage.

For instance, you can begin, *as a priority*, to focus on your own physical relaxation. Attempting to do whatever techniques or massage strokes you do, in as relaxed a way as possible. **Attempt to keep the focus within yourself and not displaced outside yourself on the receiver. Remain present in your hands and feel what is underneath them.** Breathe deep and slowly into the belly and repeatedly relax your pelvic floor and perineum. Use your body weight to achieve depth instead of muscular strength. This means your arm should be straightened at the elbow, not bent. When the arm is bent the force goes out the elbow and you end up pushing on the body with your muscles, which completely changes the quality of touch – it is a bit forced and hard. When you align lower arm and upper arm through the elbow, you become able to lean your body weight on the person, which is a relaxed force that simply moves through the other person's body. This completely changes the quality of touch and makes it very easy for the other person to receive and welcome your touch.

All these small shifts of focus will lead you to your inner world and to your being, and will come through your touch. Your massage will become more flowing and fluid and you will enjoy it more, which is a big plus. You yourself will feel enriched and nourished. You will soon begin to observe how your inner focus changes the 'how' of your touch and what that contributes to the other person's experience. I noticed that the more I relaxed my physical body, and remained totally present in my hands, the more the other person was able to dive very deeply into themselves. They found a place of simple blissful profound rest within themselves that was deeply healing and refreshing.

In my view the genitals and sexual stimulation or titillation have nothing to do with a tantric massage. There is nothing basically wrong with doing this (consciously) but it generally leads in the direction of excitement and tension that takes a person toward their circum-ference, and away from relaxing into their center. **A tantric massage should be one that encourages the receiver to relax into the core of their body, and ultimately through this inner focus,**

they become able to expand beyond their physical boundaries, which is pure bliss. Blissfulness is the experience of feeling at one with existence, floating as light as a feather, in total harmony with everything that is. And it is in *this* space that healing, integration and regeneration happens.

As mentioned earlier, if you read my books about making love doing so will perhaps help you to grasp more easily what I am suggesting in the way of tantric principles. Then see how you can apply them to massage. **Tantra is interested in 'how' a person does something, not what they do. And the how is to do whatever you do with increasing awareness.** This quality will naturally transform your touch, and give rise to elevated experiences. Wishing you many joyful hours of exploring tantra through giving massage.

Love, Diana

6. Accepting and loving my body

Dear Diana,

I just finished your book *The Heart of Tantric Sex* and I wish it would just continue. Exactly in the way you describe it, I can imagine making love. Especially when you are a bit older and you no longer find your partner 'hot', there has to be more, another level – as you say, more depth.

There is something I missed in your book. I am already fifty-four years old and after twenty-eight years of marriage my husband left me, and my two girls, for a younger woman. I went through a difficult time, letting go; the hurt had to heal and the two girls were shaken in every aspect, so that of course also affected me.

Now, after one and a half years I have fallen in love with a man of the same age as me. But now I am very self-conscious to be naked in front of him. You have to know, I am very thin, my breasts are very small (luckily there are push-up bras) and my whole body as well as my skin is not that firm anymore! **I would** have liked to read an article in your book about how to deal with age, the changes etc. and with a new partner. Only ten years ago I might probably have had less of a problem with it. Now I am already a bit in the menopause. I still have my menstruation but not regularly anymore. I would prefer to stay in the dark with him!

Nevertheless, I would find it beautiful to have eye contact during making love as you suggest in your book. I have not yet talked about this directly with my partner. I believe that he expects more under the 'packaging' and I could not bear it if he is completely disappointed! What do you advise me?

Love, Vera

Dear Vera,

It is lovely to hear that after all the challenges you have had to face, that you again have been given the possibility to open in love. This is truly healing for you. **Regarding your insecurities about your body, I suggest that you talk about your fears to your new partner. Expressing what you feel about your body will bring relaxation for you.** And it is likely to touch your partner's heart; he too is probably in a similar situation – not feeling confident about his own body. Did you ever meet a person that is totally satisfied with their physical appearance? There is an unfair emphasis on looking beautiful and eternally young. Most women will face issues around body acceptance at many points during their lives because of the perfect ideal that we are hypnotized and dominated by. And therefore as each person ages insecurity and doubt can accompany the changes. However, true beauty has nothing to do with external appearance, and so has little to do with physical ageing. True beauty resides within, and shines through the body, as the light and radiance of joy and love.

My suggestion is that you shift your focus from an objective view of your body, to a subjective view of it. This is the basic orientation of the tantric approach. All the richness lies within. Become increasingly interested in your *inner* body and your cellular sensitivity. This is where beauty lies. Be loving toward your own body, accept it, respect it, massage it, and treat it as the greatest of friends. As you begin to make love in a new way, as suggested in my book, your body will also start to change. And it does not matter that you are fifty-four. Great changes are still possible at any age, the body is always totally ready to co-operate with your awareness. Breasts grow, thighs slim down, a unity exists in the body, quality of serenity arises, movement becomes graceful, all as reflections of self- love and inner beauty. I wish you the courage to trust in your inner world, and the readiness to take steps into the unknown. Doing so will increase your joy and zest for life, which in turn will make you feel youthful and uplifted and empowered.

Love, Diana

7. I am missing my ecstasy

Dear Diana,

We visited one of your retreats some years ago. Afterwards we practiced this more gentle kind of making love for almost half a year. We both liked it very much. Since then we have started to practice very seldom and when we do, I do not feel so much in my vagina. About twice a week we have hot sex with orgasm. **I am still madly keen on my orgasm and that makes it hard for me to make 'cool' love. Nevertheless, we try making cool love now and then because I also have more and more difficulties with having a traditional orgasm.** Again and again I read your books in order to be inspired by a new way of making love.

I have also already received several vaginal massages from women. I am in a vaginal massage group and I still have the feeling my vagina is insensitive except if I stimulate my clitoris and then get hot. Then I have good sensations in my vagina. My partner would like to have more cool sex than hot sex; orgasm is not that important to him. At the moment I do not know what to do any more. **For years, sex has been the most important issue and I did almost everything for it. I read everything, did**

training's etc. And still my sexuality does not flow the way I would like it. I have stress with orgasm; I feel insecure and often I do not feel sexual desire. Then I read again about ecstasy in your book. Where is my ecstasy?

Love, Heather

Dear Heather,

Ecstasy arises in a cool environment and not a hot one. Sensitivity is the way to ecstasy, and not stimulation. So in reality you are longing for something but not creating an environment that invites it. The situation, put simply, is that you are caught in a strong sexual conditioning about orgasm. Just like almost everyone else. Sex as we know it is all about building up energy and then discharging it. There is another style and another way, and it is this window that we open for you during the seminar. But making a change does need committed and regular practice. And as you say, you only practiced about half a year, and since then very seldom.

Our basic teaching is one of awareness. Becoming aware when you are focused on the goal of orgasm, how tense the body gets, and how sensitivity is reduced. When you notice these aspects you begin to relax the body, and that allows energy to spread instead. You have to use your awareness to catch the conditioning/goals/expectations and gradually begin to move away from it. It is a process and does not happen instantly. You will eventually reach a point that you begin to forget about orgasm because being in the here and now is fulfilling.

It is difficult to have hot sensational sex most of the time and then, now and then, ask for sensitivity when you have cool sex. If you begin to relax away from orgasm in general then your vaginal tissues will become soft and sensitive. Nothing is wrong with you; the conditioning of normal sex is just very simply deeply ingrained in us – in the mind as well as in the cells.

Your ecstasy lies underneath this superficial layer. You cannot demand ecstasy and nor is ecstasy something that can be turned into a goal. You have to create an atmosphere that invites ecstasy, through presence, awareness, and relaxation. But the first step is to begin to challenge the addiction for hot sex. If you relax more into your female energy then you will find that your sensitivity interest in making love increases.

The vaginal massages that you have been giving and receiving do have a certain value, but when you have a man in your life to make love with, then the penis (with its healing qualities) is the very best way to go. The head of the penis is a powerful catalyst and is designed to do very deep resensitizing, softening and healing of the vagina.

Love, Diana

Dear Diana,

I can hardly imagine forgetting about orgasm. I also have a great longing for hot sex. To leave all this behind and to simply relax almost creates stress again. At the moment I try to relax more and to stimulate my clitoris less which also always draws me towards orgasm. And still at some point I desperately want to go for orgasm. I seem to have no choice. We can massage and touch each other and I can be simple and present, but as soon as the genitals are included I am drawn towards orgasm. It takes a lot of effort to make cool love because I only feel so little. I don't know if I can be patient enough to practice so long but I will try!

Love, Heather

8. Making rules and concepts out of tantra

Dear Diana,

After some time of practice we recognized that we have taken tantra like a new concept with rules, instead of being present and aware of what is happening. **We started thinking that it is necessary to avoid sexual attraction, excitement, orgasm and always cooling down instead of awareness and spontaneity.** On the other hand, although we are more than twenty years together, we still feel great sexual attraction between us and like very much being together in lovemaking. So we started being together in a more relaxed way, without concepts, just watching and enjoying. We continue to make love with open eyes, at times communicating what is actually happening, breast caressing, sensitive penetration, and spending much time after coming in meditative and loving space. We feel much calm and happiness in this period.

Love, Jacob & Irene

Dear Jacob & Irene,

Thank you for writing and sharing how things have been evolving since we met. It is nice to hear that you have had such a deep insight and have now found a relaxed way to be with tantra.

Yes, there is a great tendency to turn tantra into rules and a fixed concept; even though this is something that we again and again emphasize that people *should not do*. Often people get the idea that tantra is a kind of technique that means only stillness and non-movement, but this is incorrect. Tantra is alive and juicy and you will find that movements with awareness are qualitatively different to mechanical ones. **Tantra is more interested in awareness and creating love; it is not a special technique.** Stillness and non-movement is only one option and it is by no means the whole picture.

It is good to watch the mind and how it likes to do everything in the 'right' way, but this will cause tension and lack of spontaneity and will decrease your joy of exploration. Transforming the sexual energy into a meditative force is an organic living process, one to be enjoyed and celebrated. All the best to the two of you.

Love, Diana

9. My fiancée is like a virgin, her vagina is very tight

Dear Diana,

My fiancée and I bought your book *Tantric Orgasm for Women* and it helped us so much in understanding about sex and love. I am having difficulties implementing the tantric sex in my life. We live in Brazil but in different states, so we date each other one weekend in a month. My fiancée is like a virgin: her vagina is very tight and she says she can't stay for a long time having sex. She avoids positions that cause high pressure in the vagina and often we don't change position; the starting position is kept all the way through sex. Her vagina presses my penis so much and because she can't stay too long in sex, it we remain doing the traditional style of sex. When she says her time is 'ending', she or I increase the speed and I ejaculate.

I would like your help in what we can do to change this situation.

Love, Edgar

Dear Edgar,

Thank you for your e-mail and sharing your situation with me. Yes, it is not so easy to keep up a tantric exploration when you are living apart and at some distance. On the other hand, when you see each other less often you will probably be more present to each other, more aware of each other and sensitive. So in this sense being apart can have definite advantages because presence and sensitivity are tantric keys that make a great contribution to any sexual exchange.

It is quite common these days, and perhaps it has always been so, that many women do experience persisting pain upon penetration. The reasons for this are many; however, I do not wish to go into these factors now. What is more important to say is that the situation can be healed and you should read the chapters on the healing potential of sex. I suggest you read this together so that you both know what you are doing, and why you are doing it. There will need to be an atmosphere of sincerity and compassion so that healing between the penis and vagina is encouraged. It may take a while for the vaginal tissues to relax and restore, so you will both need to be patient.

And also be aware that at times old unexpressed feelings from the past can begin to flow out of the body/system. This is positive and healing and any such feelings should be given expression and not repressed. The chapter on emotions gives valuable information on how to handle old feelings/emotions, and how to keep love clear of the influence of the past.

I would also suggest for a period of time that you and your wife do not push yourselves into orgasm/ejaculation when you get the impression (or your wife tells you) that she has had enough sex and wants to stop. Instead just relax together and be inside her, until your penis relaxes and slips out of her. Keep eye contact during this time, breathe into the belly, be simple and present in your body, present to the actual moment, and let things unfold organically. I do hope these few words are of some support to you.

Love, Diana

10. Less erection due to prostate disturbance

Dear Diana,

For a while we have not in been in contact with you, and we would like to share with you what has been happening for us this year. At the end of the last year I started feeling a lack of erection during our tantra lovemaking and after the blood examination a rather high PSA (prostate gland tumor marker) was shown (more than 20). After a two-month antibiotic therapy the doctors suspected a prostate tumor, but after a biopsy no cancer cells where found. Still the PSA is high and erection is unstable.

In the beginning we thought that tantra could perhaps cause the lack of erection and tightening of prostate gland because the ejaculation was often stopped. But we also felt emotional problems caused by this situation: our fears and insecurities come to the surface. Iris felt very insecure about my love and she imagined that I maybe would like to be with other women so this caused many hard times between us. I was also not sure what was happening, so sometimes I also thought that maybe she should put something more sexy on or something like this.

At this moment we don't know whether it is an age problem (I am sixty years old) or maybe a physiological problem with the prostate gland (although doctors mentioned just urinary symptoms connected with this PSA and I do not have any urinary symptoms at all). All this is very strange so please if you can help us somehow, we would be very grateful to hear from you!

Love, Mark & Iris

Dear Mark & Iris,

Sorry to hear that you have been having health problems since we last saw you in October. The very good news is that the biopsy is clear, and the best way forward now is to be positive in attitude, and send your prostate gland all the love and light in the existence.

Mark, when a man is sixty years old, with a sexual life and history of probably close to fifty years, of which only two and a half years have been devoted to tantric exploration, it is not possible to point to tantra and wonder if it is perhaps responsible for your disturbances. With so many previous years of accumulated tensions through high levels of sexual excitement, and perhaps through masturbation too, these elements form the greater part of the picture. Who knows, perhaps the tantric practice has healed an aspect that might in other circumstances have caused greater problems? As you know, the disturbance rate of prostate in men is extremely high and getting higher.

With regards to erection, this is a subject that we go into in some depth during the course. It is a basic theme and we explain about the difference between an erection achieved through excitement and stimulation, and a spontaneous erection that can arise within the vagina itself. When there is loss of erection in any circumstances, instead of trying to deny what is happening we advise that you find a way of falling into acceptance, and to give yourself a chance to feel the feelings accompanying the loss of erection. When you relax into these feelings, allowing tears of helplessness or frustration or whatever, then this is profounding cleansing and healing on a cellular level. There will also be a corresponding shift in your psyche and attitudes.

You definitely have the tools to deal with the situation and we would suggest that you continue making love in as relaxed a way as possible and whenever possible.

We do, right from the outset of the basic lovemaking retreat, say clearly to men that nothing is wrong with ejaculation; what we simply ask them to take a look at the habit of it. And we definitely say that men *should not repress their ejaculation*. If ejaculation is pressing, better is allowing it to happen rather than forcing it to stay in the body.

Our guidelines are to rather stay in a cooler zone where ejaculation is not an issue, and if it becomes urgent at any point then you do. This point is fundamental to our tantra teaching, and we say it again and again. Repressing ejaculation and the high levels of excitement that accompany it is not great for the prostate, because tension is being added to tension.

Love, light and best wishes for your health.

Diana

11. Sexual satisfaction in spite of prostate tumor

Dear Diana,

Tracy and I participated in your Making Love Retreat in July 2009. Full of thanks, we again and again remember what you gave us in this seminar and in your books – and it is this gratitude I just want to show you and share with you today.

Maybe you remember that I couldn't or wasn't fully able to have an erection because my prostate had been removed (five years ago) due to a tumor in the prostate and the neighboring nerves. We now practice the 'soft union' by entering without erection, as you suggested, as often as possible and at least daily. Being together in this way has become something so wonderful and close. These experiences nourish our love anew until today.

However, I have to confess that at one point I often do not follow your advice to stay cool. It is always 'just heaven' to feel the vagina of my beloved so intensely that I sometimes still have an orgasm myself. I feel it in my whole body and it is very beautiful. Tracy also enjoys to feel my ecstasy. It is a very close and loving feeling for her. Then I massage her now and then with a lot of time in a tantric way. We both also love it very much when I can caress her with my tongue and she then enjoys her orgasm. So there is no imbalance between us.

Of course we again and again report to many couples with whom we are acquainted about our experience with you and recommend your books and seminars.

Love, Ian

Dear Ian,

Thank you so much for writing and sharing your love and joy in making love. And it is particularly impressive and encouraging because of the earlier limitations due to your medical condition. Congratulations for being able to devote time on a daily basis to making love! **I find frequency is a great asset in exploration and the organic unfolding of the experience. To me it sounds like you are following our advice perfectly if you continue to enjoy intensity, because what we offer are tools not rules.** The basic key is awareness. As you have heard said in the seminar many times, it is not what you do but how you do it. In this way sex is transformed into love, through using the awareness. So your experience of the love between you increasing is the outcome of the awareness that you are bringing into your lovemaking, whatever your choices or preferences along the way are. So everything is moving in a perfectly beautiful way and I am very happy for you both.

Love, Diana

12. Your tantric perspective is different

Dear Diana,

I have just begun to put your books into practice on my own, since I received them two days ago, and I am so enjoying tapping into my magnetic, feminine self and bringing this quality into my daily life as much as I can – that is an art. I love the simplicity and the depth of your exercises.

The work you do resembles the foundation of the movement work that I study and teach, so it is very satisfying to apply what I know through this into the sexual arena with your expert guidance. You are the tantra teacher I have been looking for, for two decades. I luckily have had an awesome movement teacher for the last decade, but she doesn't focus on sex, though she acknowledges that the work is tantric in its essence. I am so grateful that I have found you. You are the first tantra author/teacher I have found that I resonate with. (Although I did enjoy *Tantric Quest* by Daniel Odier, but he doesn't teach as directly as you do.)

Your emphasis on relaxation, non-technique, mind-body is so incredibly effective and immediate. I am curious where the so-called root lock and all the technical stuff comes from that I see in most tantra books and teachers. I know there are ancient texts that seem rather technical but it seems like it inhibits the essence of tantra – at least for me. Or perhaps you offer your approach for those who do not resonate with the 'structured' approach – the more paths the merrier?

Your approach is more feminine, perhaps and, just like the movement work, isn't for everyone, I suppose. My sense, actually, is that you, like my movement teacher, have tapped into the underlying universal principles of tantra and are teaching from a fluid, feminine perspective that has guiding principles but isn't mired in technique. I'm guessing that these ancient arts originated from a fluid, feminine pool of wisdom and that in order for men to understand it, they choose to break it down into techniques, like yoga, and make it all more linear and structured. I'm sure that was very useful on some level for men, perhaps!

But that beneath all of that structure, there is still an essential energetic you have to access in order to really grasp the essence of tantra. And, it seems, women are the ones that can tap into that and teach it first. So thank you! Although, you mention two male teachers who influenced you! So, there goes my argument. Anyway, if I never get to witness you in person, at least I have your very well written books! Many thanks.

Love, Sharon

Dear Sharon,

Thank you writing and sharing your perception of the tantric domain, and it certainly sounds like your movement work and my approach are one and the same thing. As you say, there are some underlying guiding universal principles that can be accessed in a number of ways. Thank you too for sharing your evaluation of my work, the appreciation, and the encouragement.

A great deal of what exists in the field of neo-tantra, as I see it, does not represent the essence of tantra. As you say, there is an emphasis on the technical side of tantra, but for me the enquiry has always been – am I doing or being? And I kept going in the direction of 'being', using the body as a bridge to the present and cellular aliveness and vitality. In this way one arrives in the being where lies the source of love within each one of us.

To me this essence represents the difference between tantra and the Taoist sexual practices. Tantric sexual practice falls under the umbrella of spirituality and meditation and has roots in India. While Taoist sexual practice falls more under the umbrella of health and medicine and has Chinese roots. In this way the orientations are very different. Through tantric sexual practice-increased health and vitality is a by-product, it happens anyway, it is not the focus. Tantra is more interested in awareness, relaxation and meditation. Taoist sexual practices will usually have distinct goals to the different techniques, ways to move energy around the body that involve 'doing' something. So the whole basis is effort, and therefore tension. So from the roots upwards they grow into very different flowers.

Perhaps at advanced stages of Taoist practice one is naturally led into the spiritual world of relaxation, meditation and the present. However, for less experienced practitioners there will usually be a desired outcome or goal in the future, that prevents the capacity to be here and now, the essence of meditation.

So the whole orientation and basis have different points of departure, and that is why for me all the techniques naturally fall away. Because at the base usually there is a goal or a doing, no matter how subtle it may be. It's not a relaxation into the here and now and the innate intelligence of the body. **Bliss arises in an environment of egolessness, naturalness and timelessness, so it is a matter of getting out of the way and melting into what 'is' on a cellular level.** And in my experience, the Taoist 'energy-locking' type of phenomena happen by themselves, when the time is right, and without effort or doing but in pure presence, and perhaps a handful of times only, as part of the evolution and transformation of sexual energy as it relaxes, comes into balance and rises through the system. And indeed, perhaps this is the actual root of the Taoist techniques. **Inner energy events happened naturally to people when they were in a certain state of being, and then afterward the happening is taken and developed into a technique, one that has now become separated from its roots and true environment.**

Interesting your comment about the feminine. And yes, I did receive the guidelines from two rare and precious male masters, Osho and Barry Long. I put their different insights into direct action, filtered the information through my body for a number of years, and was then able to understand things from a totally different perspective. One thing that is absolutely clear to me is that it is *only* because of these two very excellent sources that I found myself in the field. I had absolutely no goal, only curiosity about sex. I just happened to end up where I ended up. And I owe it to my sources, nothing else. I was surprised when I first begun to work (almost twenty years ago) in Europe and other parts of the world that people would say how 'different' my approach was, but I myself had no idea that I had landed up in a completely other domain of experience to the usual neo-tantra approaches.

I will tell you what I heard Osho once say: that really only a woman is able to teach tantra. So in that sense your observation is very astute. It took me a long time to understand why this is so, but now I do. Woman is the space, she is the container, and she can influence the environment and anyone who moves through it. For me right from the start I found it completely easy to create an environment that enabled people to relax into their essential elements. It is no effort at all; I can do so blindfolded if I wish. In January 1993 in India, I taught my very first group of five couples and I was stunned that 'it' worked immediately, from the very first moment. People slipped effortlessly into an altered dimension – it was truly magical. And just through a handful of simple keys that I had distilled over a period of years. I just 'knew' how to go about it because I had managed 'it' thousands of times within myself. I do recall an assistant I had at that time asking me if this was really the *very first* time I had guided people because it seemed to be so easy and natural. To her it seemed I had always been doing it.

Barry Long, as you know, made the revolutionary audio lectures called *Making Love*. However, he himself never created the space for people to have sexual experience under his guidance. I think in a way he did not know how to create the environment for the people. He had the knowledge and information without a doubt, but not how to transmit it to people when you have them together for a period of time. I heard that once he said that for a teacher to teach tantra to a group of participants the teacher would have to make love with each of the participants! Well, such is not my understanding and experience.

For a short period of time many years ago I had a lover who had once been a close assistant of Barry Long's. And he kept asking me again and again, how do you do it? Meaning how do I manage my weeklong Making Love Retreats. He said he could not imagine how the practical information could be put into action in real life with a group of couples.

You may be interested to get hold of the CD of the guided breast meditation for women that Michael and I put out last year. It is called *MaLua Light Meditation* and there you will find a groundbreaking quote from Osho, who says that for women *all meditation should start at the breasts*. He says that most meditation techniques are developed by man and they are therefore suitable for men, but not for women. He gives a meditation exclusively for women - to melt and merge with the breasts because they are the route to higher orgasmic experiences and the awakening of kundalini energy in women.

Thank you for giving me the opportunity to get this all down in writing. I was touched by your sensitivity and clarity. Best wishes for each day.

Love, Diana

13. Relaxation and menstrual purification

Dear Diana,

It is already two weeks since we finished the Making Love Retreat. Until now I can still feel the nice relaxation in my body. It is as if I have fallen deeper into my body. It feels sheltered and cozy. I also feel that my ego doesn't like it very much and this part of me can't believe that it's just about relaxation and not about doing and thinking of a thousand things at a time. Sometimes it is hard to stay out of this mindset and to stay in touch with my body and the deeper parts of myself.

It is also great to feel more closeness, love and respect towards my partner. We make the time to connect our genitals each day for a short period and once a week we make a date for a long lovemaking. Most of the times it's very special and it touches my heart deeply. Sometimes though it can be hell when it doesn't work the way we want.

I also feel a lot of things happening in me. Before my last menstruation I felt completely emotional and very puffed up, like a lot of stuff wanted to come out. Also the bleeding was very dark and clotted, also painful. I had to laugh about you saying that things such as pre-menstrual syndromes (PMS) will reduce, because for me it has been quite a lot worse than normal. But I'm sure it is a process that just has to happen.

In a way it feels a bit scary that my partner feels more close to me than ever. Of course it is great but I feel more fear coming over the possibility of losing him and that can bring up insecurity in me. Despite this I would never change or stop with the things we have started through your course! It feels like a spiritual journey together to grow in love and consciousness and that is the path where my heart wants to go.

Love, Wendy

Dear Wendy,

Thank you so much for the heart-warming sharing and we are grateful that you allowed the teachings to touch your hearts and beings. And the best we could possibly wish to hear is that you are managing to make love each day!

As far as the menstrual syndromes getting exaggerated, as I understand it, this is usually part of the natural healing cycle. Things somehow have to get a little bit worse in order to get better. The presence of dark and clotted blood usually represents part of the cleansing and purification that takes place when there is a change of lovemaking style. Through the relaxation and awareness, old congestion moves out of the system on physical and emotional levels.

Dark clots may happen a couple of times or so; however, if you feel there is *any* room for concern, please do consult a doctor. I myself had the same clearing, and many women have reported something similar to me. As a guideline, if the blood is dark (old) then all is probably well. If the blood is fresh, and continues to remain fresh for a while, then consult a doctor.

I can understand your fear about the possibility of losing your partner and how it can bring up insecurity. Perhaps to remember Osho's words in your moments of insecurity will be of support – fear is the absence of love. So whenever you feel fear coming up then remember that love is the medicine for fear. Fall into your body, relax into your being, and connect with the source of love in yourself. In this simple way you can help to prevent fear getting the upper hand and disturbing your love. Best wishes to both of you.

Love, Diana

14. Tantra without a partner

Dear Diana,

For more than ten years, I have been longing to participate in one of your Making Love groups but it never happened because of my partner who I was with for over twenty years. And now I am in a very new relationship and this man is also not really open to do the group. Making love is my real nature; it was always like this in my inner experience. What can I do with you without a partner?

Love, Carol

Dear Carol,

There is a great deal you can do for yourself as an individual, and without necessarily coming to participate in a group with me. I can only give you impulses, but in the long-term the effort will have to be yours. Many guidelines and keys are given in all of my books and these can be put into immediate effect. **In fact, tantra starts with you and your body, learning to use it as a bridge to the present, relaxation and awareness. This can be done in ordinary daily activities. The basics do not apply to sex alone, but also to the body in general.**

I suggest you read *Tantric Orgasm for Women* where there are many meditations to increase femininity and the awareness of the inner world. When the atmosphere around and within you changes, through your own awareness, there can be an alchemical effect on the partner, as they too sense a different quality in the air. This will subtly change them and create more presence and awareness. In particular it is suggested to meditate on your breasts for about a half hour every day so as to anchor you in your positive energy-awakening pole. At its base, tantra is individual work, not couple work. The individual comes before the couple, so you can start to work on yourself in a variety of ways and observe how the intensity of your awareness transforms any given moment. Perhaps in time your partner will change his thinking. All the best.

Love, Diana

15. Healing the pain and shame of sexual abuse

Dear Diana,

I write this report on my experiences for you as part of your ongoing research into sex. To be able to describe the profound experiences during the Making Love Retreat, I have to go back a bit. Six years ago, when I was seventeen, someone I knew forced me to have sex with them. I endured it several times. This was my first experience of sexuality. Never before in my life was I that ashamed. From then on somehow I thought it normal for sex to be only painful, for the woman to swallow the sperm and for my body not to be okay as it is. I did not have a sexual relationship for a long time afterward and I felt very uncomfortable in my body. At times I even hated it.

Two years later I got to know my partner, Tom. With him everything proceeded more slowly and I felt understood and cared for. Sexuality, however, was still very difficult for me. Even though Tom never pushed me to do anything or demanded anything from me during all this time I felt under pressure. **I felt responsible for his sex life, for his orgasm. I always felt pain but I never dared to say anything because I thought it was my problem and I was ashamed. I thought I was the only one who could not enjoy sexuality. Rarely had I enjoyable sensations. And I was ashamed about this also.**

As long as I can recall, however, I imagined sex to be

something wonderful. Something that connects two beings, lets them melt together! Something very close to life, to our being, to our existence. Something spiritual, and empowering. And even though I knew that Tom was thinking the same way and that our love was more important to him than his orgasm I was very burdened by all the expectations and dogmas regarding sexuality.

At some point the longing for something else, however, grew. This feeling that there had to be more was very strong. I started therapy and I tried to come to terms with the past. There were times when I could enjoy sexuality and did not have pain. And still afterward I often lay besides Tom and I felt used and empty. Used by him – he who loves me so much! I tried this way a lot, but I was never happy with it and this issue also challenged our relationship again and again.

When I was twenty-one, I read the book *Tantric Orgasm for Women* by Diana Richardson. I touched me deeply and liberated me very much. Now I finally knew why my body had reacted in this way. And I could see another way to go! Tom and I experimented a lot with the book and we had very beautiful experiences. But still somehow I had the feeling that I could only understand the true essence of Diana and Michael's teaching by attending a seminar with them. And so we attended the seven-day seminar.

From the first day on I felt very well in my body. The daily exercises, meditations and the dancing were very good for me. I could listen to very fine movements in my body and my inner attention grew enormously. I was looking forward to the exercises and the meditation with great joy, and it was as if a whole new world had opened up before me. The world of my wonderful body! Even so, the first two times we made love were still a hard test for me. I had strong pain at the entrance of the vagina and I was very sad about it. I had had a lot of expectations regarding the seminar and through the pain I again connected with the depth of all my painful feelings and experiences. Then Diana recommended us to self-massage the whole pelvic area.

On the third afternoon I was lying next to Tom and first I did a solar plexus massage and then the recommended self-massage. Next to the entrance of my vagina I discovered several very painful places. It tried to relieve the pain with massage. Doing that, I felt sick and I could not breathe. I tried to stay with this feeling and to release everything. The whole energy went up to my head. Then we tried the soft penetration without erection and afterward I realized that Tom's penis was massaging exactly those painful places. This was such a liberating insight!! That afternoon I cried often. Many pictures of the rape surged but I was so present and caring with my body that I simply could let go of them.

One thing that helped me a lot during this week was the concentration on the breasts. I had done the guided *MaLua Light Meditation* (CD) for women before the seminar, but it seems to me be that only during the seminar I really realized the significance of the breasts. In the night after the first time when we focused on the breasts, I had a dream. I saw my breasts very clearly and felt a lot of love for them. In the dream, I had a child and I breastfed it and saw milk coming out of my breasts. I can still remember the dream vividly.

From then on, I found it delightful to be with my attention fully in my breasts. Every time after a short while there was a response from my vagina in the form of a pulsation, a streaming or a feeling as if a door slowly opened.

One evening of the seminar, we did a pelvic massage. Many feelings came up and afterward it was very difficult for me to be close to Tom. I was confused and full of emotions. Only much later during the evening mediation I realized that in fact it had brought us together much more. I could feel the opening and let Tom in without pain. It was an overwhelming feeling that I cannot express in words. It is as if his penis touched my heart!

Now I know that the pain is not my enemy but my friend. The fear of sex falls away completely because we can simply lie there for two hours and softly penetrate millimeter by millimeter. The feelings that come up do not scare me and I can see this rape in a completely different light. I am reconciled with it. For viewing and living lovemaking in such a different way is a gift bigger than anything that has ever happened to me before.

I think that we both discovered our true qualities during this week. In our relationship, we are standing at a very different point now. The issue of emotionality has contributed to this a lot. It was often in our way. Now I am also sure that through it my genitals often tensed up. Awareness and humor have taken the place of arguments, discussions and emotions. Regular lovemaking brings us closer but – and this is important – it also brings me closer to myself.

Two weeks have passed now since the seminar. Before, I could not imagine that so many things would change in such a short time. I meditate with the *MaLua* breast meditation every day. Not because I think I have to, but out of sheer joy. During the meditation I can feel a connection from my breasts to my toes. It is wonderful! Tom and I make love frequently. The pain that I had for many years at the entrance of my vagina is gone. Completely gone! This is like a miracle to me. Sometimes I still feel pain in others areas in the vagina and sometimes we are not as present as we intended. Often emotions come up and for some time I feel very sad. But we both feel that this is our way and it feel great to learn more about it. **In my life I could not imagine to have so much joy with sex. Without being excited, and (almost) without expecting anything. Just to be in the here and now, and to feel the love. There is so much love awakening – it extends beyond my relationship with Tom. There is so much gratitude and love towards the whole existence.**

Since we have practiced this kind of lovemaking, a physical detoxification process is underway. Especially my teeth, skin and the whole head seem to be purifying. Also my inner world seems to want to get rid of something. Many emotions come up and I am hypersensitive to sound and touch. This makes it sometimes hard to be relaxed and without expectations during making love. Tom's love and patience, however, help me very much.

One more thing that is very important to me: All aims and all striving for something far distant, future plans etc. are gone. (Even though I am a person who loves to plan.) Vanished into thin air. I think about the seminar every day, the radiance and the words of Diana and Michael, Osho's quotes and my own inner being that slowly blossoms. **I no longer have the need to become something because now I know that I am something.**

In my training as a midwife I have seen many stories. Stories of women who were not allowed to be women. I saw traumatic births and strained bodies and souls. It hurt me each time to see it. **Hardly any woman trusts or loves her body. In the Making Love Retreat I learned a lot also regarding midwifery. How much more conscious and loving giving birth could be if there were more consciousness, love and trust!** How much more gently the new beings could be welcomed on earth! I also think that the knowledge about the 'inner magnet' and the significance of the breasts could have a decisive influence to the process of birth. Personally I think that giving birth cannot be separated from sexuality and therefore I would be happy if the ancient knowledge, the original trust and the teaching of Diana and Michael could be given to many couples and if one day it would also find its place in midwifery.

How much more peaceful, loving and fulfilled would the world be with this way of making love and living! Thank you, Diana and Michael!

Love, Judith

Dear Judith,
We are deeply touched by your sharing of your profound inner

process. Thank you so much for taking the time to put your insights and healing experiences into words. It acts as a great gift of encouragement for others to know that sexual energy can be embraced and used as a healing, integrating and empowering force.

Blessings to you both, and thank you for your sincerity.

Love, Diana

16. I would like to educate and show others

Dear Diana,

Do you offer workshops to train (certificate) people in your technique, so they can teach this as well, or be a sexual healer? *I loved Tantric Orgasm for Women.* It speaks to me. **For the first time someone has explained what my body needs.** I would like to educate and show others.

We have done some of the exercises in your book. The other day he decided to try something during sex, and I am going to be blunt with you. He sucked on my nipple while entered in me and orgasmed. I felt this electric circle, even though I had not orgasmed myself while he was in me, but something had profoundly changed. The intimate circuit was tender, ignited an energy, flowing from my breasts, his mouth, his penis, my vagina, my heart, opening for us both, to the point that while he orgasmed I saw his eyes roll up in his head and he went into an altered state. We were both blown away in the process. The circling of Love Energy between negative and positive poles was amazing. Thank you for bringing this to the world, and to my life.

Love, Shelley

Dear Shelley,

It is a joy to hear my book resonated within you and has explained what your body needs. What is most beautiful is that you are open and receptive to seeing and feeling your body in a completely new way.

Nice to hear of your groundbreaking experiences, and the image of your partner's eyes rolling up in his head makes me smile - I can well understand!

I appreciate your sincerity and wish to educate and share this approach with others. But no, in answer to your question, we do not offer a teacher training that will qualify others to teach. **The situation is a delicate one in that to convey a new understanding as a 'teacher'; one needs to have gone through a process of self-exploration and transforming one's own sexual energy. So it is not simply a matter of passing on some acquired information and techniques, but creating a whole shift in consciousness within you as an individual. And as a couple.** And this can only be achieved through personal exploration and tantric practice of some years. If a couple come to us and express an interest in teaching, *after* they have participated in several of our workshops, *and* been practicing for several years, then for sure we are more than happy to support them and prepare them to become teachers of our work. For these reasons we do not offer teacher trainings per se.

Love, Diana

17. Love is a by-product of a rising consciousness

"Love is a by-product of a rising consciousness.
It is just like a fragrance of a flower.
Don't search for it in the roots; it is not there.
Your biology is your roots;
Your consciousness is your flowering.
As you become more and more an open lotus of consciousness,
You will be surprised - taken aback –
With a tremendous experience which can only be called love.
You are so full of joy, so full of bliss;
Each fiber of your being is dancing with ecstasy.
You are just like a rain cloud that wants to rain and shower.
The moment you are overflowing with bliss,
A tremendous longing arises in you, to share it.
That sharing is love."

Osho, Life's Mysteries

Appendix: Complete List of Letters

Chapter 3: Emotional Aspects

Chapter 4: Sexual Subjects

Chapter 5: Special Issues

Books and Resources

Book References

Richardson, Diana. *The Heart of Tantric Sex*. O Books, 2002 (First edition published as *The Love Keys – The Art of Ecstatic Sex*, 1999).

Richardson, Diana. *Tantric Orgasm for Women*. Destiny Books, 2004.

Richardson, Diana & Michael. *Tantric Sex for Men – Making Love a Meditation*. Destiny Books, 2010.

Richardson, Diana & Michael. *Tantric Love – Feeling vs. Emotion: Golden Rules to Make Love Easy*. O Books, 2010.

Richardson, Diana. *Slow Sex – The Path to Fulfilling and Sustainable Sexuality*. Destiny Books, 2011.

Further Reading

Osho. *From Sex to Super-Consciousness*. New York, St Martin's Press, 2003. Osho. *Tantra: The Supreme Understanding*. India, The Rebel Publishing House, 1998.

Osho. *The Book of Secrets 1-5*. New York, St Martin's Press, 1998.

Long, Barry. *Raising Children in Love, Justice and Truth*. Barry Long Books, 1998.

Long, Barry. *Making Love: Sexual Love the Divine Way*. Barry Long Books, CD.

Long, Barry. *Love Brings All to Life*. Barry Long Books, CD.

Robinson, Marnia. *Cupid's Poisoned Arrow: From Habit to Harmony in Sexual Relationships*. North Atlantic Books, 2009.

Rosenberg, Marshall. *Nonviolent Communication: A Language of Life*. Puddle Dancer, 2003.

Additional Resources by Diana & Michael Richardson

Richardson, Diana & Michael. *MaLua Light Meditation for Women* – Innenwelt Verlag, Cologne, 2008. CD (Guided breast meditation with music).

Richardson, Diana with Michael. *Time for Touch – Massage, Awareness, Relaxation.* – Innenwelt Verlag, Cologne, 2010. DVD. (Instructions for full body massage).

Richardson, Diana. *Making Love–What you always should have known about Sex.* Innenwelt Verlag, Germany, 2010. DVD Live Public Talk.

All resources are available from
www.livingloveshop.com

'The Making Love Retreat'
with Diana and Michael Richardson
www.livinglove.com

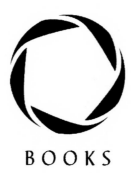

BOOKS

O is a symbol of the world, of oneness and unity. In different cultures it also means the "eye," symbolizing knowledge and insight. We aim to publish books that are accessible, constructive and that challenge accepted opinion, both that of academia and the "moral majority."

Our books are available in all good English language bookstores worldwide. If you don't see the book on the shelves ask the bookstore to order it for you, quoting the ISBN number and title. Alternatively you can order online (all major online retail sites carry our titles) or contact the distributor in the relevant country, listed on the copyright page.

See our website **www.o-books.net** for a full list of over 500 titles, growing by 100 a year.

And tune in to myspiritradio.com for our book review radio show, hosted by June-Elleni Laine, where you can listen to the authors discussing their books.

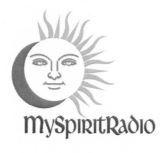